Psychopharmacology Supplementum 1

# Sleep, Benzodiazepines and Performance

## Experimental Methodologies and Research Prospects

Editors:
I. Hindmarch H. Ott T. Roth

With 81 Figures

Springer-Verlag
Berlin Heidelberg New York Tokyo 1984

Dr. Ian Hindmarch
Human Psychopharmacology Research Unit, University of Leeds
GB-Leeds, LS2 9JT

Dr. Helmut Ott
Research Laboratories, Section Electrophysiology/Psychometrics, Schering AG
P.O. Box 65 03 11, D-1000 Berlin 65

Professor Dr. Tom Roth
Sleep Disorders and Research Center, Henry Ford Hospital
Detroit, MI 48202, USA

Library of Congress Cataloging in Publication Data
Main entry under title:
Sleep, benzodiazepines and performance.
(Psychopharmacology supplementum; 1)
Papers presented at a workshop during the VII. International Congress of Psychiatry in Vienna, 1983.
Bibliography: p. Includes index. 1. Insomnia-Chemotherapy-Congresses. 2. Benzodiazepines-Congresses. 3. Insomnia-Research-Congresses. I. Hindmarch, I. (Ian), 1944 –. II. Ott, H. (Helmut). III. Roth, T. (Tom). IV. Series. RCS48.S53 1984 616.8′49 84-5309

ISBN-13: 978-3-642-69661-9 e-ISBN-13: 978-3-642-69659-6
DOI: 10.1007/978-3-642-69659-6



Typesetting: Daten- und Lichtsatz-Service, 8700 Würzburg

2125/3140-543210

# Preface

The following papers were presented at an International Workshop on experimental methodologies and research strategies in sleep, benzodiazepines and performance during the VII. International Congress of Psychiatry in Vienna 1983. Authors were asked to examine and review the methods used and the results obtained from the various studies within their particular expertise and to provide guidelines for future strategies in the psychopharmacology of sleep.

It has long been felt by sleep researchers, psychopharmacologists and clinicians that the effects of drugs on sleep or even sleep itself cannot be evaluated without reference to the daytime behaviour of the individual. Sleep and daytime performance are complementary aspects of the same circadian cycle. The modification of sleep parameters by hypnotic medication must necessarily have an impact upon daytime behaviour.

The overall change in a patient's daytime behaviour following nocturnal administration of a benzodiazepine is of importance when considering the tolerability and safety of the drug in clinical use. Alterations to the integrity of daytime performance also have consequences for that patient's subsequent sleep and nocturnal behaviour.

Thus this workshop was conceived as a platform for examining the interrelationship of sleep, benzodiazepine hypnotics and daytime performance from pharmacological, psychological, experimental and clinical standpoints. The following papers also highlight the complexity of the interaction between sleep, patient, drug and daytime performance and emphasize the need to approach problem areas with appropriate research strategies and experimental methodologies.

*I. Hindmarch H. Ott T. Roth*

# Contents

**Differential Effects of Benzodiazepines**



**Résumé**

# Sleep and Insomnia

# Polysomnographic and MMPI Characteristics of Patients with Insomnia

F. Zorick, N. Kribbs, T. Roehrs and T. Roth[1]

**Contents**



**Abstract**

This report represents the polysomnographic aspects of sleep and the psychological characteristics of a large series of patients with insomnia classified according to the diagnostic system of the Association of Sleep Disorders Centers. The findings for patients in the various diagnostic categories were compared to those of symptomatic patients with no objective findings. 9 specific diagnoses were made, but 4 diagnoses accounted for the majority of patients. The 4 most prevalent were psychophysiological disorders (15%), psychiatric disorders (17%), nocturnal myoclonus and restless legs (18%), and no objective findings (19%).

Patients of a sleep disorders center are a select population and may not be representative of the general population of patients with insomnia complaints. The psychological characteristics of the different diagnostic groups were assessed by computing the number of elevations on the MMPI. Patients with a psychiatric diagnosis exhibited the highest number of MMPI elevations, as might be expected. Patients with nocturnal myoclonus had the lowest number of elevations. The other groups did not significantly differ from the group with no objective findings. Polysomnographic measures of sleep differed considerably among the diagnostic groups. The groups with medical disorders, respiratory impairment, atypical polysomnographic features, and nocturnal myoclonus had similar short sleep latencies to those of the group with no objective findings. With longer wake times before sleep and significantly different from patients with no objective findings were the psychophysiological disorder, psychiatric disorder and drug and alcohol groups. Patients with a circadian rhythm disturbance had the longest latencies. Time spent awake after sleep onset was high and significantly different from the no objective findings group in patients with a psychophysiological disorder, psychiatric disorder, restless legs syndrome and nocturnal myoclonus diagnosis. The circadian rhythm disturbance group was the only group without increased wakefulness during sleep. Overall, there were large differences in the total sleep time of the groups. Finally, quality of sleep as measured by percent stage 1 showed the greatest number of significant differences compared to patients with no objective findings.

---

1 Sleep Disorders and Research Center, Henry Ford Hospital, Detroit, MI 48202, USA

Psychopharmacology Supplementum 1
Editors: I. Hindmarch, H. Ott and T. Roth

**Key Words**

Diagnostic classification system/Differential diagnosis/ECG/EEG/EMG/EOG/MMPI/Nocturnal myoclonus/Polysomnographic findings/Psychiatric disorders/Psychological characteristics/Restless legs/Sleep disorders centers.

# 1 Introduction

The importance of the differential diagnosis of insomnia complaints has become very evident based on the accumulated experience of clinicians at sleep disorders centers. To address the problem of differential diagnosis of insomnia the Association of Sleep Disorders Centers published the first diagnostic classification system for disorders of initiating and maintaining sleep (Association of Sleep Disorders Centers 1979). In an earlier report we applied the association's classification system to a series of patients with insomnia (Zorick et al. 1981). We reported polysomnographic findings for different diagnostic groups based on comparisons to normal volunteers. However, there was a small number of patients in each of the diagnostic categories making it important to replicate the previous findings. Additionally, in that series we found a group of symptomatic patients (no objective findings) who had normal sleep; they did not differ in polysomnographic aspects of sleep from the asymptomatic controls. These symptomatic, but normal sleepers, are a more appropriate comparison group.

This report presents the polysomnographic aspects of sleep and psychological characteristics of a large series of patients with insomnia who were classified according to the association's diagnostic system. Findings for patients in the various diagnostic categories were compared to those of symptomatic patients with no objective findings.

# 2 Methods

## 2.1 Subjects

The subjects of this report are 199 patients, 96 women and 103 men, at the Henry Ford Hospital Disorders Center who were evaluated for their complaint of difficulty initiating and maintaining sleep (DIMS). Most were referred by a physician and all patients had had their sleep problem for a minimum of six months.

## 2.2 Procedures

Before the initial clinic visit each patient completed a questionnaire detailing the history and symptoms of their sleep complaint. Each also provided a two-week sleep diary of their usual sleep habits. During the clinical interview the sleep history was reviewed, a medical and psychiatric history taken, and a physical and mental status examination was given. The Cornell Medical Index and the Minnesota Multiphasic Personality Inventory (MMPI) were also completed.

Seven days before undergoing a polysomnogram all sedative medications were discontinued. Use of other medications, including diuretics, antihypertensives, digitalis, and tricyclic antidepressants, within seven days of the polysomnogram were allowed if clinically indicated. 28% of patients in this series had used one of these medications prior to the polysomnogram.

At least one all-night polysomnographic evaluation was obtained from each patient. The polysomnogram included the standard central (C3) and occipital (Oz) electroencephalograms (EEGs), electrooculogram (EOG), submental electromyogram (EMG), and electrocardiogram (ECG) recorded with a V5 lead. In addition airflow was monitored with oral and nasal thermistors and leg movements with electrodes placed over the right and left tibialis muscles. All recordings were scored for sleep stages according to the standards of Rechtschaffen and Kales (1968). Respiration recordings and tibialis EMG recordings were evaluated by a clinical polysomnographer (Guilleminault 1982).

Each patient then received a specific diagnosis derived from the Association of Sleep Disorders Centers Diagnostic Classification of Sleep Disorders (Association of Sleep Disorders Centers 1979). This diagnosis, based on the results of the entire clinical evaluation including the interview, questionnaires, and nocturnal polysomnogram, was the consensus diagnosis of three clinical polysomnographers. Each patient in this series received a single diagnosis that accounted for the full spectrum of signs and symptoms observed. Comparisons among diagnostic groups were made using analyses of variance and post hoc t-tests and the chi square where data were nonparametric.

## 3 Results

### 3.1 Relative Prevalence

The prevalence of different diagnoses at this center is presented in Table 1. Nine specific diagnoses were made, but four diagnoses accounted for the majority of patients. The four most prevalent were psychophysiological disorders (15%), psychiatric disorders (17%), nocturnal myoclonus and restless legs (18%), or no objective findings (19%). Within each diagnostic group the distribution of men and women was even except for the drug or alcohol use, respiratory impairment, and nocturnal myoclonus groups which were about two-thirds male.

**Table 1.** Relative prevalence of diagnoses

| Diagnoses | *n* | % of Total | % Male |
|---|---|---|---|
| Psychophysiological disorder | 29 | 15 | 48 |
| Psychiatric disorder | 35 | 17 | 50 |
| Drug or alcohol use | 13 | 7 | 69 |
| Sleep-related respiratory impairment | 15 | 8 | 73 |
| Nocturnal myoclonus and restless legs syndrome | 36 | 18 | 58 |
| Medical disorder | 12 | 6 | 50 |
| Circadian rhythm disturbance | 11 | 5 | 64 |
| No objective findings | 38 | 19 | 42 |
| Atypical polysomnographic features | 10 | 5 | 40 |
| Total | 199 | | |

Patients of a sleep disorders center are a select population and may not be representative of the general population of patients with insomnia complaints. Therefore, the prevalence of any specific diagnosis in this series cannot be considered representative. This is due to the specific entry criteria and referral sources used by a given center. For example, in one national survey the percentage of insomnias caused by psychiatric disorders varied from 4 to 67 at different centers (Coleman et al. 1982). Additionally, the sex distribution at this center is biased for men in comparison to national surveys of the general population where women predominate (Karacan et al. 1976). Moreover, elderly patients are underrepresented in this series relative to the well-documented increased incidence of sleep complaints among elderly people (Roehrs et al. 1983). Table 2 presents the distribution of specific diagnoses in elderly (age 61 or greater) compared to nonelderly patients. The predominant diagnoses among elderly differed from that of the nonelderly. Most often elderly had an objective basis to their complaint (i.e. few no objective finding diagnoses) compared to nonelderly ($X^2 = 4.67$, $p < 0.05$). More often in the elderly the cause was not a psychiatric disorder ($X^2 = 5.53$, $p < 0.02$). Typically, for elderly it was nocturnal myoclonus and restless legs disorders ($X^2 = 10.06$, $p < 0.001$) or drug or alcohol use ($X^2 = 6.79$, $p < 0.01$).

**Table 2.** Diagnoses in elderly and nonelderly

| Diagnoses | ≤ 60 years | | ≥ 61 years | |
|---|---|---|---|---|
| | *n* | % | *n* | % |
| Psychophysiological disorder | 22 | 14 | 7 | 15 |
| Psychiatric disorder | 32 | 20 | 3 | 6[a] |
| Drug or alcohol use | 6 | 4 | 7 | 15[b] |
| Sleep-related respiratory impairment | 13 | 9 | 2 | 4 |
| Nocturnal myoclonus and restless legs syndrome | 20 | 13 | 16 | 33[b] |
| Medical disorder | 7 | 5 | 5 | 10 |
| Circadian rhythm disturbance | 10 | 6 | 1 | 2 |
| No objective findings | 34 | 22 | 4 | 8[a] |
| Atypical polysomnographic features | 7 | 5 | 3 | 6 |
| Total | 151 | | 48 | |

[a] $p < 0.05$; [b] $p < 0.01$

## 3.2 Psychological Characteristics

Psychological characteristics of the different diagnostic groups were assessed by computing the number of elevations on the MMPI (a T score greater than 70 on any clinical scale). Mean number of MMPI elevations for each group are presented in Table 3. The number of elevations varied considerably among the specific diagnostic groups. As might be expected, patients with a psychiatric diagnosis had the highest number of elevations, significantly higher ($t = 2.5$, $p < 0.01$) than patients with no objective findings. Patients with nocturnal myoclonus had the

**Table 3.** MMPI elevations

| Diagnoses | Mean | SEM |
|---|---|---|
| Psychophysiological disorder | 2.1 | 0.42 |
| Psychiatric disorder | 4.3 | 0.55 |
| Drug or alcohol use | 3.1 | 0.60 |
| Sleep-related respiratory impairment | 1.4 | 0.37 |
| Nocturnal myoclonus and restless legs syndrome | 1.0 | 0.36 |
| Medical disorder | 3.0 | 1.18 |
| Circadian rhythm disturbance | 2.7 | 1.06 |
| No objective findings | 2.8 | 0.45 |
| Atypical polysomnographic features | 2.1 | 0.60 |

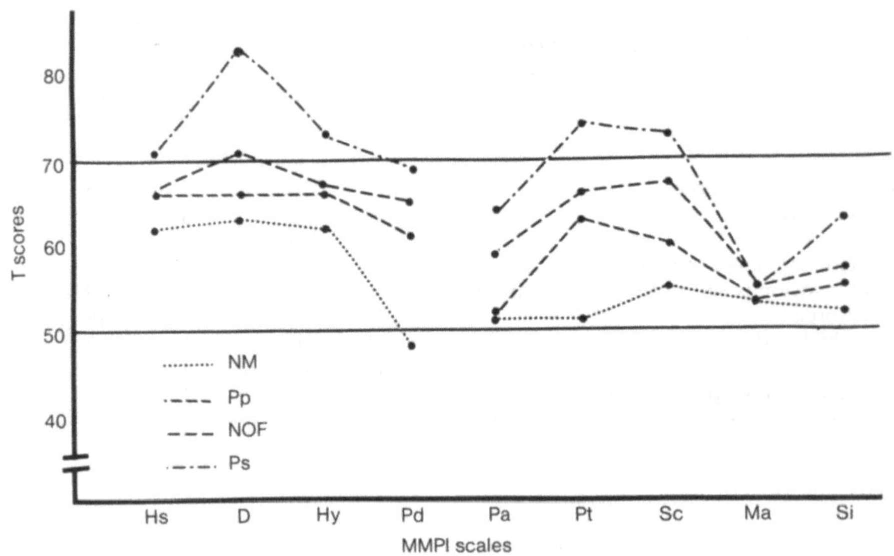


**Fig. 1.** MMPI elevations in the four most common diagnostic categories. *NM* nocturnal myoclonus, *Pp* psychophysiological disorder, *NOF* no objective findings, *Ps* psychiatric disorder

lowest number of elevations, significantly lower ($t = 3.1, p < 0.002$) than patients with no objective findings. The other groups did not differ significantly from the group with no objective findings. One note of caution, the higher means found for patients with circadian rhythm disturbance and medical disorder diagnoses may be spurious due to the relatively small group size and the unusually high variability.

Further comparisons of the pattern of MMPI scores on each of the clinical scales were done. This analysis of the MMPI profile for the four most common diagnostic groups revealed interesting similarities and contrasts which are illustrated in Fig. 1. The profiles of patients with a psychiatric disorder, a no objective findings, and a psychophysiological disorder diagnosis were all quite similar. Each group had the same high and low scales, varying only by degree. In contrast, patients with a nocturnal myoclonus diagnosis had a relatively flat profile. Interestingly, this group is relatively older than the other groups.

### 3.3 Polysomnographic Characteristics

Polysomnographic measures of sleep differed considerably among the diagnostic groups. First, patients differed in their ability to fall asleep (see Fig. 2). Wake time before sleep was 14 min for the patients with no objective findings. The medical disorder, respiratory impairment, atypical polysomnographic feature, and nocturnal myoclonus groups had similar short sleep latencies and did not differ from the no objective findings group. With longer wake times before sleep and significantly different from patients with no objective findings were the psychophysiological disorder ($t = 2.79$, $p < 0.01$), psychiatric disorder ($t = 2.35$, $p < 0.02$), and drug and alcohol ($t = 2.22, p < 0.03$) groups. Patients with a circadian rhythm disturbance had the longest latencies, 64 min, and differed significantly from the no objective findings group ($t = 2.42$, $p < 0.01$).

The ability to maintain sleep differed among the diagnostic groups also and is illustrated in Fig. 3. Time spent awake after sleep onset was high and significantly different than the no objective findings group in patients with a psychophysiological disorder ($t = 2.80$, $p < 0.01$), psychiatric disorder ($t = 2.10$, $p < 0.04$), restless legs syndrome ($t = 2.23$, $p < 0.05$), and nocturnal myoclonus ($t = 3.80$, $p < 0.01$) diagnosis. The medical disorder, respiratory impairment, atypical feature, and drug and alcohol groups were also elevated, but did not

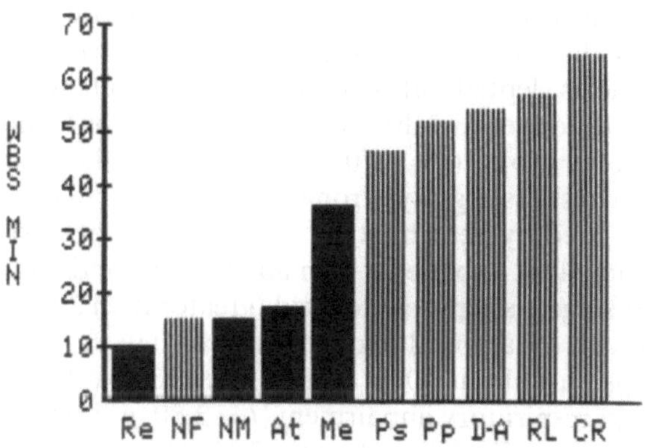


**Fig. 2.** Minutes of wake time before sleep in the various diagnostic categories. Groups with striped bars are significantly different from the NF (no objective findings) group. *Re* respiratory impairment, *NM* nocturnal myoclonus, *At* atypical polysomnographic features, *Me* medical disorder, *Ps* psychiatric disorder, *Pp* psychophysiological disorder, *D–A* drug and alcohol use, *RL* restless legs syndrome, *CR* circadian rhythm disturbance

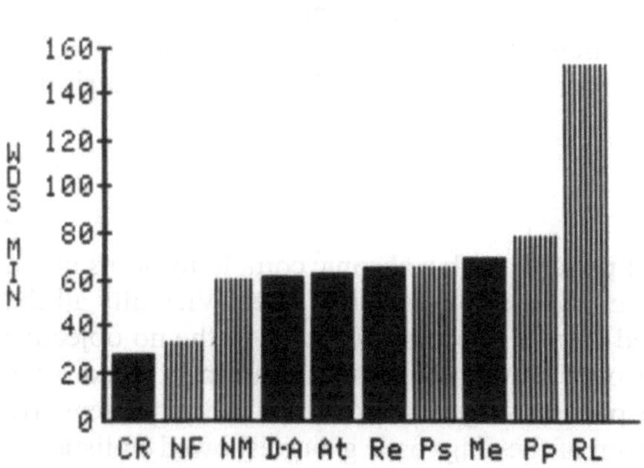


**Fig. 3.** Minutes of wake time during sleep in the various diagnostic categories. Groups with striped bars are significantly different from the NF (no objective findings) group. All diagnostic groups are identified in the legend of Fig. 2

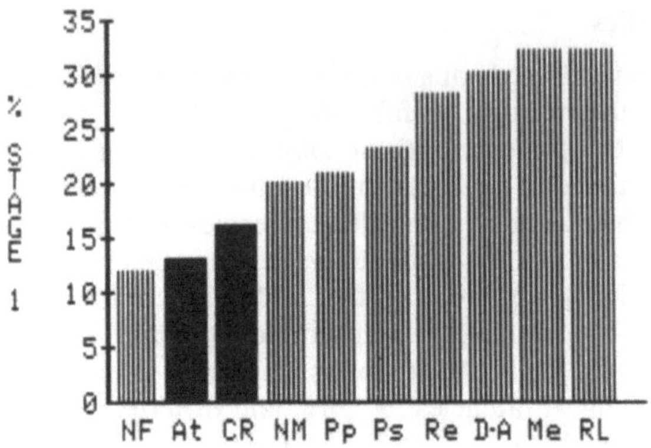


**Fig. 4.** Percentage of stage 1 sleep in the various diagnostic categories. Groups with striped bars are significantly different from the NF (no objective findings) group. All diagnostic groups are identified in the legend of Fig. 2

differ significantly from the patients with no objective findings. The circadian rhythm disturbance group was the only group without increased wakefulness during sleep. The only patients awakening earlier than scheduled were those with a psychiatric disorder; they differed significantly from patients with no objective findings ($t = 4.80$, $p < 0.01$).

Overall, then, there were large differences in the total sleep time of the groups. Compared to the patients with no objective findings who slept for 7.4 hours, patients with a psychophysiological disorder ($t = 5.10$, $p < 0.01$), psychiatric disorder ($t = 4.90$, $p < 0.01$), medical disorder ($t = 2.70$, $p < 0.01$), and drug or alcohol use ($t = 4.1$, $p < 0.01$) diagnosis slept about two hours less. Patients with nocturnal myoclonus slept somewhat longer (6.5 h) than these groups, but still shorter than the no objective findings group ($t = 3.70$, $p < 0.01$). The shortest sleepers (4.2 h) were patients with restless legs syndrome ($t = 3.86$, $p < 0.01$).

Finally, quality of sleep as measured by percent stage 1 showed the greatest number of significant differences compared to patients with no objective findings. This is illustrated in Fig. 4. Percent stage 1 sleep was elevated (greater than 20%) for all the groups except patients with an atypical features or circadian rhythm disturbance diagnosis. Four groups had about 30% stage 1 sleep and differed from the no objective findings group: respiratory impairment ($t = 2.80$, $p < 0.01$), drug or alcohol use ($t = 3.5$, $p < 0.01$), medical disorder ($t = 3.18$, $p < 0.01$) and restless legs ($t = 3.50$, $p < 0.01$). With a little over 20% and differing from the no objective findings group were patients with nocturnal myoclonus ($t = 2.8$, $p < 0.01$), psychophysiological disorders ($t = 2.50$, $p < 0.01$), and psychiatric disorders ($t = 2.80$, $p < 0.01$).

## 4 Discussion

The results of this study show that patients with a chronic complaint of insomnia do in fact show polysomnographic evidence of disturbed sleep. Virtually all the diagnostic groups showed elevated stage 1 sleep as compared to the no objective findings group. Most of these groups also showed an elevation of wake time during sleep. Yet it is noted that percent stage 1 seems to be the more sensitive measure of sleep maintenance. Seven of the diagnostic groups showed statistically

**Table 4.** Significant[a] polysomnographic parameters by diagnostic category

| Diagnoses | WBS | WDS | WAS | % 1 |
|---|---|---|---|---|
| Atypical polysomnographic features | | | | |
| Medical disorder | | | | + |
| Sleep-related respiratory impairment | | | | + |
| Circadian rhythm disturbance | + | | | |
| Drug or alcohol use | + | | | + |
| Nocturnal myoclonus | | + | | + |
| Restless legs syndrome | + | + | | + |
| Psychophysiological disorder | + | + | | + |
| Psychiatric disorder | + | + | + | + |

[a] $p < 0.05$ compared to no objective findings group

significant increases in stage 1, while only four of the groups showed significant increases in wake during sleep. This disparity between percent stage 1 and wake during sleep may reflect the fact that patients with chronic insomnia complaints often show multiple arousals during sleep. These arousals typically result in a "lightening" of sleep, shifts to stage 1 sleep, but do not result in actual awakenings.

The other major finding of this study is that the pattern of sleep disruption seen in the various diagnostic categories is different (see Table 4). Some groups show no sleep disturbance, some only a sleep induction or maintenance problem, and some show both. The atypical polysomnographic findings group showed no evidence of sleep disruption at all. The only consistent finding in these patients was an intrusion of alpha activity into NREM sleep. This finding has been associated with the insomnia complaint of patients with fibrositis syndrome (Moldofsky et al. 1975). With some evidence of disturbed sleep was the circadian rhythm disturbance group (predominantly phase delay syndrome; Weitzman et al. 1981), who showed only a long sleep latency with otherwise normal sleep. Patients with restless legs also had a long sleep latency, but unlike circadian rhythm patients also showed sleep fragmentation after sleep onset. The other three groups with prolonged sleep latencies as well as sleep fragmentation were psychophysiological, psychiatric, and drugs and alcohol. It is interesting to note that these groups have a behavioural or psychogenic component to their sleep problem. One might speculate that people with fragmented sleep will develop a moderate "sleep debt" and as a result, have an increased tendency to fall asleep. However, with the addition of a behavioural component to the insomnia, this tendency to fall asleep quickly as a result of the "sleep debt" is overridden. This speculation is supported by the fact that some patients show sleep fragmentation without a behavioural component to their insomnia. These patients (medical, respiratory impairment, nocturnal myoclonus) have normal sleep latencies.

Finally, the present results show that psychological evaluations alone are not adequate to determine the etiology of a sleep complaint. Most diagnostic groups show at least some MMPI abnormalities. In many cases, this may not be the cause of the problem, but rather the consequence of having a chronic medical condition. There have been reports of MMPI abnormalities in patients with other medical conditions (Spergel et al. 1978). In addition, we found some diagnostic categories with no MMPI abnormalities. Thus, in dealing with patients with insomnia, a careful psychiatric and sleep evaluation is needed to determine the underlying cause of the problem.

In addition to clarifying the differential diagnosis of insomnia, these results also have important implications for treatment. The identification of specific causes of insomnia underscores the necessity of treating the primary cause and not the symptom. If the insomnia is secondary to a psychiatric or medical condition or a sleep-related physiological abnormality (e.g. apnea, nocturnal myoclonus), the underlying condition and not the symptom should be treated (Zorick et al. 1981; Roth and Zorick 1983). Similarly, in patients with an insomnia complaint but no polysomnographic evidence of disturbed sleep, symptomatic treatment is not indicated. Symptomatic treatment may be considered in patients with documented persistent insomnia only when no specific primary cause can be identified or when no specific treatment for a particular condition is available (e.g. nocturnal myoclonus). In terms of evaluating the efficacy of symptomatic treatment (i.e. sedative hypnotics), these data would suggest that key efficacy parameters are often overlooked. We found that stage 1 sleep was a sensitive index of a patient's ability to maintain sleep. Often the effects of drugs on stage 1 sleep are not reported. Percent stage 1, and in fact, arousals leading to stage 1 may prove to be the polysomnographic parameter which best correlates with patients' perception of efficacy.

## References

Association of Sleep Disorders Centers (1979) Diagnostic classification of sleep and arousal disorders, 1st edn. Sleep 2:21–57

Coleman R, Roffwarg H, Kennedy S, Guilleminault C, Cinque J, Cohn M, Karacan I, Kupfer D, Lemmi H, Miles L, Orr W, Phillips E, Roth T, Sassin J, Schmidt H, Weitzman E, Dement W (1982) Sleep-wake disorders based on a polysomnographic diagnosis – a national cooperative study. JAMA 247 (7):997–1003

Guilleminault C (ed) (1982) Sleeping and waking disorders: Indications and techniques. Addison-Wesley Publishing Co, Menlo Park, CA

Karacan I, Thornby J, Anch M, Holzer C, Warheit G, Schwab J, Williams R (1976) Prevalence of sleep disturbance in a primarily urban Florida county. Soc Sci Med 10:239–244

Moldofsky H, Scarisbrick P, England R et al. (1975) Musculo-skeletal symptoms and non-REM sleep disturbances in patients with fibrositis syndrome and healthy subjects. Psychosom Med 37:341–351

Rechtschaffen A, Kales A (eds) (1968) A manual of standardized terminology, techniques and scoring system for sleep stages of human subjects. NIH, Bethesda, MD

Roehrs T, Zorick F, Sicklesteel J, Wittig R, Roth T (1983) Age-related sleep-wake disorders at a sleep disorders center. J Am Geriatr Soc 31 (6):364–370

Roth T, Zorick F (1983) The use of hypnotics in specific disorders of initiating and maintaining sleep (insomnias). In: Chase M, Weitzman E (eds) Sleep disorders: Basic and clinical research. Spectrum Publications, New York, pp 255–264

Spergel P, Ehrlich G, Glass D (1978) The rheumatoid arthritic personality: A psychodiagnostic myth. Psychosom 19 (2):79–86

Weitzman E, Czeisler C, Coleman R, Spielman A, Zimmerman J, Dement W (1981) Delayed sleep phase syndrome: A chronological disorder with sleep-onset insomnia. Arch Gen Psychiatr 38 (7):737–746

Zorick F, Roth T, Hartse K, Piccione P, Stepanski E (1981) Evaluation and diagnosis of persistent insomnia. Am J Psychiatry 138 (6):769–773

# Issues in the Diagnosis and Treatment of Insomnia [1]

W. Dement, W. Seidel and M. Carskadon [2]

**Contents**



1 This research was supported by NIA grant number AG 02504, Dr. William Dement is supported by Research Scientist Award number MH 05804 from NIMH

2 Stanford University, Sleep Laboratory, School of Medicine, Stanford, CA 94305, USA

Psychopharmacology Supplementum 1
Editors: I. Hindmarch, H. Ott and T. Roth

**Abstract**

Most people attribute a restorative function to sleep. This is because experimental or clinical sleep disturbance is usually followed by annoying symptoms of fatigue and sleepiness the following day. Can these daytime changes be documented objectively? In the past several years, the Multiple Sleep Latency Test (MSLT) has been developed and validated as an objective quantitative measure of sleepiness. Multiple assessments of sleep latency yield a profile of sleepiness across the day. This profile changes in the predicted direction with acute total and partial sleep deprivation, chronic sleep deprivation, sleep satiation, and in comparisons between hypersomnia patients and controls.

Sleep and wakefulness are complementary phases in the daily cycle of human existence. Adequacy of sleep and energetic wakefulness next day are interacting phases in this cycle. Insomnia can be seen as a perception of disturbed sleep with daytime consequences, but is essentially also a symptom. This paper reviews a number of issues in the diagnosis and treatment of insomnia. The dimensions, daytime consequences and longitudinal aspects of insomnia are considered. Most investigations to date have been geared towards the problem of chronic insomnia and yet we are all likely to suffer from transient insomnia at some point. Psychiatric and psychophysiological disorders have been shown to be the most frequent causes of disorders of initiating and maintaining sleep. Moreover, there is an apparent disparity between subjective and objective sleep parameters with, for example, objectively disturbed sleep in noncomplaining subjects.

The criteria of hypnotic efficacy and the effects of triazolam and flurazepam on sleep and daytime alertness have been investigated in normals, chronic insomniacs and the elderly.

In general, chronic insomniacs showed all degrees of daytime alertness regardless of nocturnal sleep parameters. About one-third could be classified as fully alert all day long in spite of their complaints. The effect of flurazepam and triazolam on sleep (improvement) was essentially the same. Daytime effects were most closely related to half-life. The long-acting benzodiazepine, flurazepam, impaired daytime alertness although nocturnal sleep was improved. Triazolam improved not only nighttime sleep but also daytime alertness.

**Key Words**

All-night clinical polysomnography/Chronic insomniacs/Daytime alertness/Flurazepam/Ideal hypnotic/Multiple Sleep Latency Test (MSLT)/Noncomplaining subjects/Pseudo-Insomniacs/Transient insomnia/Triazolam.

An adequate scientific basis for the clinical management of insomnia does not exist (IOM 1979; Dement 1982; Dement in press). One reason is the persistent tendency to regard insomnia as the root problem rather than as merely a symptom requiring diagnostic evaluation. The situation is rapidly changing, however, and progress in two key areas has provided a major impetus. The first area is experimental pharmacology including the development and marketing of new hypnotic compounds. The second area involves the practice of sleep disorders medicine which has introduced new specificity into the diagnosis and treatment of insomnia (ASDC 1979; Coleman et al. 1982b). Accordingly, the time has arrived to formulate a rational and empirical framework for dealing comprehensively with the problem of insomnia in all its forms and to utilize this framework to identify gaps in our knowledge and errors in our concepts. In this paper, we will attempt to outline several issues involving insomnia as a phenomenon, as an objective of clinical investigation, as a very important clinical symptom, and as a problem requiring therapeutic intervention.

## 1. What Is Insomnia?

The word "insomnia"is often used, but rarely defined. Webster's Dictionary says, "prolonged or abnormal sleeplessness". This use of the word conjures up a stereotypical image that is often far removed from reality. Most people who complain of disturbed sleep almost never complain of not sleeping at all. Moreover, polysomnographic determination of objective sleep parameters in patients who complain of "insomnia" often shows *apparently* normal or near normal amounts of sleep (see below). Finally, in mania or in a few exceptional people, objective sleep time may be greatly reduced in the absence of a complaint.

In terms of our current knowledge, the most consistent general definition we can formulate is that insomnia stands for all the conditions related to the perception of disturbed or inadequate sleep. How does an individual judge that sleep is inadequate? Adequacy of sleep is generally judged in one of two ways. The individual makes a direct judgement about his sleep experience, or he makes an inference about his sleep based on the way he feels in the daytime. Obviously, both may be involved simultaneously.

In summary, the condition of insomnia is a perception of disturbed or inadequate sleep. When we confront the bewildering array of sleep-related problems and the infinite series of factors, syndromes, illnesses, life conditions, and personalities that appear to be involved, however, we realize that much of what is "known" may be premature generalization. Thus insomnia is roughly analogous to pain – many kinds, many locations – a symptom with a thousand causes and associated factors.

## 2. Can We Have Insomnia Without a Daytime Consequence?

Perhaps one of the most common human experiences is a night of markedly disrupted sleep due to external factors, for example noise or a strange environment. Such a night is predictably followed by lassitude and fatigue the next day. The obvious change in behavior is usually explained to others by saying, "I didn't get enough sleep last night." Often, if the day is filled with events that are particularly exciting or associated with vigorous physical activity, this consequence does not appear to be present. Such a commonplace occurence models what we have known for decades, that acute sleep loss causes daytime sleepiness and that physical activity can offset the effects of experimental sleep deprivation (Kleitman 1963). We assume that daytime sleepiness is usually present in transient insomnia; however, there are almost no laboratory data describing objective sleep parameters in transient situational insomnia.

Let us imagine an individual who feels that his sleep is always light and restless, and that he typically wakes 10 or 20 times a night. During the day, however, he feels wide awake, ebullient, energetic, and well-rested, even when engaged in sedentary activity. *In such a case, when there is no daytime symptom whatsoever, we must consider that the amount and quality of sleep, whatever it may be, is entirely adequate.* Sleep might be regarded as inefficient – that is, the time spent sleeping does not account for most of the time in bed – but certainly not inadequate. The most obvious explanation for the inefficiency is simply that too much time is spent in bed. Such an individual might believe that everyone needs the same amount of sleep and is trying to get more sleep than he or she actually needs to be fully alert in the daytime.

Because the adequacy of sleep is often judged in terms of energetic wakefulness the next day, it is difficult to conceive of inadequate sleep when one feels "great" in the daytime. On the other hand, it is possible to conceive of a patient who "needs" very little sleep, whose only problem is the boredom or discomfort of lying awake at night, and who wants more hours of oblivion; however, it is difficult to accept that this is a legitimate medical problem. It is worth mentioning that many patients seem hesitant to complain of daytime sleepiness, anticipating, perhaps, that the doctor will say, "Well, why don't you take a nap?" When they hear such a relatively casual response, patients often feel that the doctor has not fulfilled his obligation to provide some relief if possible.

What about daytime symptoms that are not those typically associated with experimental sleep deprivation? Sleep disorders centers now have a great deal of experience with patients who have chronic or persistent insomnia. There appear to be two distinct types of chronic insomniacs, those whose daytime symptoms involve various shades of sleepiness and fatigue and those whose daytime symptoms are qualitatively different. The latter may involve anxiety, vague dysphoria, nervousness, "a band around the head," feelings of depression, impairment, irritability, and so on. The symptoms can be very troublesome, but the patient emphatically denies daytime sleepiness or any tendency to fall asleep. In addition, regardless of the specific symptom and however strange or unrelated to sleep it may seem, the patient unequivocally attributes it to disturbed sleep.

Although we are naturally skeptical when people complain that they can't sleep at night but feel just fine in the daytime, there is no *a priori* reason to exclude such instances from our comprehensive definition of insomnia. However, it should be absolutely clear that an adequate history of insomnia *must* involve a thorough inquiry about daytime symptoms and their relation to nighttime sleep. An initial denial of daytime symptoms may only mean that the patient is afraid the doctor will de-emphasize the significance of the nighttime complaint. In actual practice, daytime symptoms are frequently taken for granted when someone says, "I have trouble sleeping."

## 3. What Are the Dimensions of Insomnia?

The complaint of insomnia is heterogeneous and complex. Setting aside for the moment the issue of daytime consequences, the perception of inadequate sleep (insomnia) can have many dimensions. At one extreme, insomnia can involve only one or a few bad nights. Insomnia can be transient, with a clearly limited and relatively brief time course, or it can be chronic and unremitting. Finally, insomnia can occur as intermittent bouts of transient episodes recurring at regular or irregular intervals.

Duration is the most important aspect of insomnia. Patients with transient insomnias far outnumber patients with chronic insomnias, although the latter number in the millions. Even so, sleep disorders researchers are not too familiar with transient insomnia except in their personal lives. A patient who has had insomnia less than a week is never seen at a sleep disorders clinic and rarely seen by a general physician. Thus sleep specialists usually have no problem judging chronicity, because most of their patients claim the insomnia has been present for years. Almost no data are available on transient problems and how they present to physicians. The general impression is that the patient consults his doctor for another problem and as an afterthought says, "Oh, by the way, I'm having trouble sleeping".

Conceptually and practically, there is a world of difference between transient insomnia and chronic insomnia. Obviously, the line that divides transient and chronic cannot be specified to the nearest day; however, the transient insomnias generally last a few days to a few weeks, while the duration of chronic insomnia is usually measured in months and years.

One reason for this early discussion of transient insomnia is to remind us that we may tend to generalize from our own personal experience to all insomnia. Accordingly, certain investigators tend to feel that all insomnia is caused by excitement, anxiety, and stress. Furthermore, transient sleep disturbance, as with experimental sleep loss, appears to be associated with feelings of fatigue, tiredness, exhaustion, and sleepiness in the daytime. Transient insomnia tends to fit our time-honored notions and stereotypes about sleeplessness. There is abundant evidence, however, that the complaints of daytime consequences in chronic insomnia vary from incapacitating to none.

In addition, the specific nature of the perceived nocturnal disturbance can involve difficulty falling asleep, difficulty staying asleep, or both. When a patient attaches specific amounts to his complaints, they are referred to as "subjective sleep parameters". There are no widely accepted quantitative subjective criteria; however, most patients report longer than 30 min to fall asleep or a habitual sleep time less than 6 or 7 h. Although patients may say that they get no sleep at all, this is never true. About one patient in 70 remains completely awake all night on at most *one* of several nights during clinical polysomnography. To a degree, insomnia is probably self-limiting in much the same way sleep deprivation is self-limiting: total or partial sleep deprivation leads to extreme sleepiness, a condition that motivates the organism to obtain more sleep.

## 4. Objective Sleep Parameters in Chronic Insomnia

Are the various perceptions of disturbed sleep accurate; that is, are they exactly parallelled by changes in sleep that can be measured objectively by polysomnography? In the diagnostic classification system developed by the Association of Sleep Disorders Centers (ASDC 1979), this subjective-objective disparity is classified under the label, "Insomnia with No Objective Findings". This diagnosis is not at all uncommon, even in sleep center patient populations generally thought to reflect patients with the more severe complaints (Coleman et al. 1982b). To put this question into perspective, we might ask whether the administration of hypnotics is justified if there is a perception or complaint of disturbed sleep but no objective sleep disturbance.

Chronic insomniacs are without comparative frame of reference; that is, they do not experience abrupt change from undisturbed sleep to disturbed sleep. Nonetheless, most patients with chronic sleep complaints have very definite ideas about the inadequacy of their sleep, describing their sleep *quantitatively* as the number of minutes it takes to fall asleep, the amount of wakefulness during the night, and a specified reduced total amount of sleep; i.e., "I never sleep more than two hours," or "I almost never sleep at all". Such unreflective complaints can be refined using daily sleep questionnaires. Thus, completing a typical "morning questionnaire" in a sleep clinic, a patient with insomnia is required to state as accurately as possible the number of minutes it took to fall asleep and how long he slept on the preceding night, knowing full well that this sleep has been precisely measured. The patient is thus under some constraint with regard to exaggerating the complaint. Even under these circumstances the chronic insomniac is likely to overestimate sleep latency and nocturnal and wakefulness and to underestimate total sleep time. Normal sleepers are usually less discrepant in their subjective estimates.

Because we can measure objective sleep parameters with great precision, we are in a position to pose and attempt to answer several questions. How accurate or inaccurate are the subjective sleep parameters in chronic insomnia? Can there be a perception of disturbed sleep (complaint) when sleep is essentially normal? A mass of laboratory and screening data show that most insomniacs on most nights fall asleep in less than 30 min and sleep more than 6 1/2 h, particularly when time in bed is 8 h or longer, even though they state that they hardly sleep

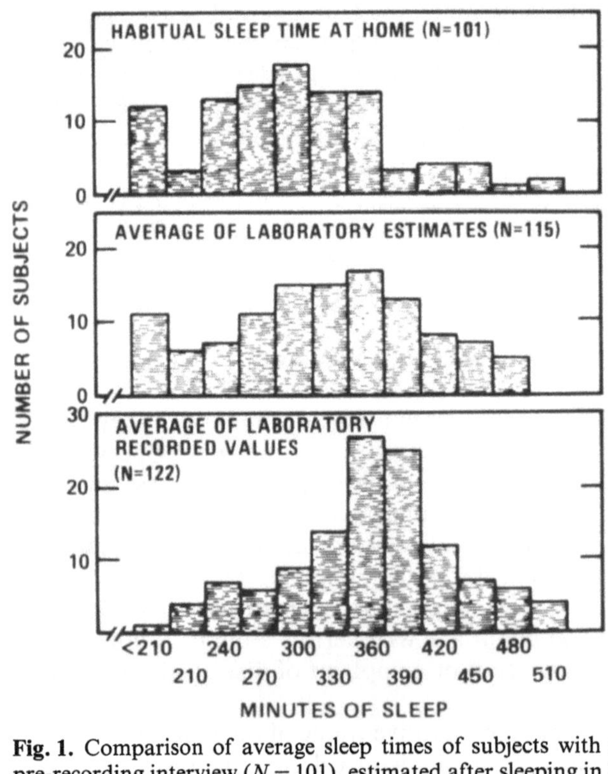


**Fig. 1.** Comparison of average sleep times of subjects with insomnia complaints reported in pre-recording interview ($N = 101$), estimated after sleeping in laboratory ($N = 115$), and recorded in the laboratory ($N = 122$). (Reprinted with permission from Carskadon et al. 1976)

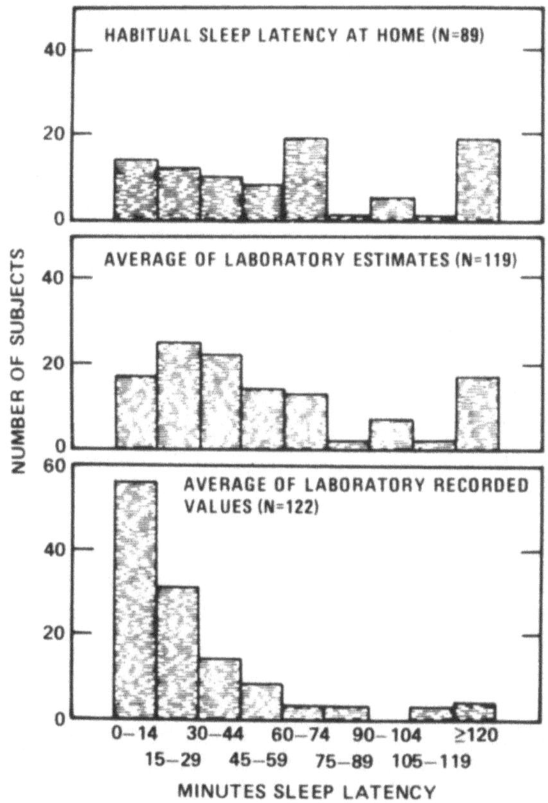


**Fig. 2.** Comparison of average sleep latencies of subjects with insomnia complaints reported in pre-recording interview ($N = 89$), estimated after sleeping in laboratory ($N = 119$), and recorded in laboratory ($N = 122$). (Reprinted with permission from Carskadon et al. 1976)

at all (Carskadon et al. 1976; Sherer et al. 1981). Figures 1 and 2 illustrate such data from a study of 122 chronic insomniacs (Carskadon et al. 1976). Conversely, can sleep be unambiguously disturbed in the absence of any complaint of insomnia?

## 5. What is Disturbed Sleep? What is Normal Sleep?

At the present time, there is no widely accepted comprehensive definition of normal sleep. To phrase it another way, there is no definition of what constitutes disturbed sleep or the critical values for sleep latency, total sleep time, and number of awakenings that would be the lower limit for disturbed sleep. If there were widely accepted standard conditions, our tendency would be to define normal sleep as the sleep that is recorded from noncomplaining healthy individuals recorded under these standard conditions. Even this definition, however, appears to allow a spectacular amount of sleep disturbance to be termed "normal".

We can imagine a sample of 45-year-old men and women monitored in a standard setting with their accustomed bedtime and sleeping until they awaken spontaneously in the morning. We might then be able to say that a normal sleep latency is 23 min, normal sleep time is 7 h 47, and there are normally 12.7 arousals. What would we then say about a 45-year-old who has exactly these normal sleep parameters yet complains bitterly of insomnia? The data that have been gathered on this issue suggest that lack of a difference in sleep parameters between complainers and noncomplainers is more the rule than the exception (Monroe 1967; Williams et al. 1972; Carskadon et al. 1976). Figure 3 schematically depicts this overlap.

There are at least three possible interpretations of a wide overlap of objective sleep parameters between normal sleepers and insomniacs. The first possibility is that the insomniac in many cases needs more sleep than normal sleepers and the complaint simply reflects this increased sleep need. The second possibility is that the complaint of insomnia is purely and simply a neurotic symptom having no relation to sleep parameters at all. For example, suppose a patient has a character disorder and is unable to participate in certain interpersonal relationships. The patient "learns" that he will be considered exempt from these unpleasant demands if he says he has had terrible insomnia the night before. The third possibility is that there is some overlooked abnormality in the sleep of the insomniac that is not reflected in standard sleep parameters, particularly as derived from the standard scoring procedures of the Rechtschaffen and Kales manual (1968). In the first and third instances, we might expect the complaint of insomnia to be associated with feelings of diminished alertness in the daytime or other symptoms clearly attributed to the perceived sleep disturbance. In the second case, the patient could be fully alert in the daytime.

A particularly important example of the third possibility is the "transient arousal." Such events have been reported by Březinová et al (1982) and Lavie et al. (1982) in COPD and nasal obstruction syndrome, respectively. Carskadon et

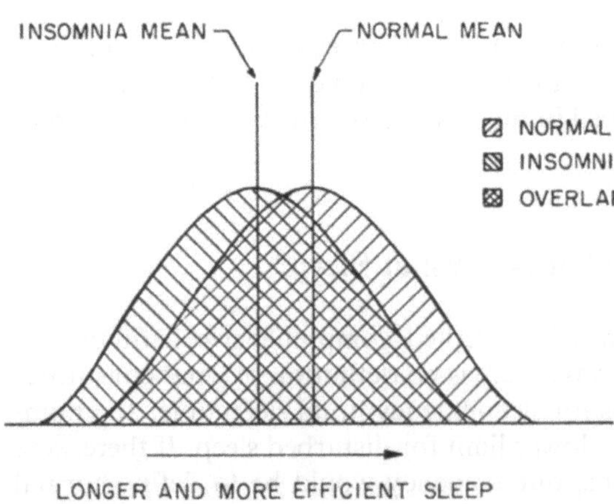


**Fig. 3.** Schematic representation comparing objective sleep times of persons with insomnia (a perception of impaired sleep) and persons with no sleep complaint. Although the means are significantly different, equally as striking is the overlap of values between the two groups

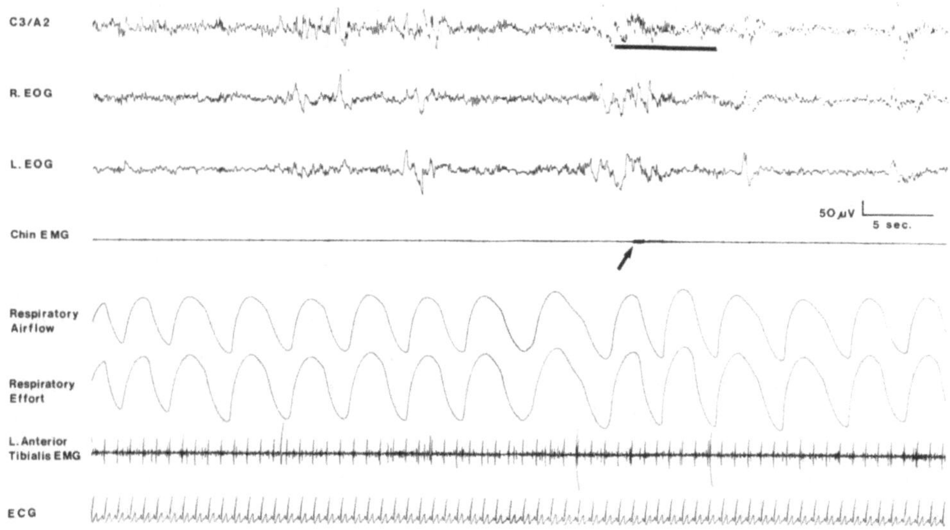


**Fig. 4.**. Recording of a "transient arousal." A brief burst of alpha in the EEG is not assessed using standard sleep-scoring criteria. Such arousals may, however, be predictive of subsequent daytime sleepiness

al. (1982a) have also reported transient (>2 >15 s) arousals in noncomplaining elderly volunteers, documenting an association between these events and daytime sleep tendency. Figure 4 shows an example of a transient arousal.

The transient arousal is only one example of a hidden sleep problem that may be associated with inadequate sleep. Moldofsky and his colleagues (1975) have described an alpha-delta EEG pattern in the sleep of patients with the "fibrositis syndrome" associated with nonrestorative sleep. Guilleminault et al. (1976a) described two occult causes of insomnia: sleep apnea and a sleep-related abnormal swallowing reflex. Nocturnal myoclonus, or periodic leg movements during sleep, appears to be a widespread phenomenon, although its relationship to the insomnia complaint is not clear at this time (Coleman et al. 1980).

If we could agree on an objective definition of normal sleep, then we could construct a paradigm to divide human sleep into four groups: 1) individuals who complain of sleep disturbance and whose sleep is objectively disturbed compared to the objective norms; 2) persons who complain and whose sleep is not objectively disturbed; 3) people, particularly in the older age groups, whose sleep is spectacularly disturbed and who do not complain; and 4) individuals, the normals, who do not complain and whose sleep is not disturbed.

In the absence of a consensus definition of disturbed sleep, we must continue to define insomnia as a complaint – a perception of disturbed sleep. Thus, anyone who has a complaint about a perceived sleep disturbance, together with a daytime consequence, has insomnia regardless of objective sleep parameters. In other words, we reaffirm the current tendency to define insomnia for clinical purposes solely in terms of the presence of a subjective complaint. The only exception is the person with a daytime complaint who says, "I must have insomnia or I wouldn't have this problem", but who does not directly perceive a sleep disturbance. (Such patients can seem fairly bizarre. For example, "I must have insomnia because my heart races. My heart wouldn't race if my sleep was better".)

In terms of the paradigm outlined above, we might ask who are the valid patients? This is not quite the same as asking, who are the insomniacs? Thus, if we saw objectively disturbed sleep and daytime sleepiness in a noncomplainer, we might feel that treatment was nonetheless indicated in order to improve daytime alertness.

Specifying the boundary between objectively disturbed and undisturbed sleep may be a problem. Early adolescents sleep through the entire night with very few awakenings (Carskadon 1982). On the other hand, individuals have been described who show hundreds of brief arousals during the night as well as substantial numbers of longer awakenings. Thus, there is no problem at the extremes in describing objective nocturnal sleep as either disturbed or undisturbed. Furthermore, we agree that the essence of disturbed sleep is fragmentation, frequent interruption, or lack of continuity. However, there has never been agreement on a quantitative definition or series of definitions of boundary conditions. That is, what are the minimal number of interruptions that would characterize disturbed sleep, or conversely, the maximal number of interruptions that could be allowed as undisturbed sleep?

## 6. Should There Be Standard Conditions for Assessing Insomnia?

When patients complain of either transient or persistent insomnia, we have an interest in the actual nature and degree of the sleep disturbance. This concern is of even greater relevance in chronic insomnia, in which we are interested in comparing what the patient says with what he does. In addition, it is important to compare the objective sleep parameters of chronic insomniacs with those of age- and sex- matched control subjects. In order to make such a comparison, we must define the standard conditions of the sleep recordings and be sure the standard conditions are applied to both groups.

At the present time, widely accepted sleep recording standards have not been specifically adopted by the sleep research community. For example, should a subject go to bed at a prearranged time which is sometimes designated mainly for the convenience of the laboratory staff, or should the subject keep a log and go to bed at the time he habitually goes to bed at home? Subtle factors surrounding the bedtime ritual can easily prolong sleep onset – noise, comments by technicians that heighten anxiety, and so forth. How many hours should be spent in bed? Should the patient get out of bed at a prearranged laboratory time? Should he be awakened and thus interrupt the spontaneous sleep period? Or should the subject be allowed to sleep *ad libidum* however long it is, even though this means that time in bed cannot be held constant? Parenthetically, if an insomniac has to be forceably awakened and dragged out of bed at a predesignated time every morning, he may be incurring chronic partial sleep deprivation as a result. When the subject awakens in the morning with the feeling that he has had enough sleep, how is the decision to terminate the time in bed actually made? Sleep recordings can be affected by the way in which all of the foregoing are specified.

Another exceedingly important issue in standardization is the number of nights that should be required under standard conditions to yield an adequate characterization of the nocturnal sleep of a single individual. Most investigators agree that one night is insufficient due to the likelihood of a "first night effect" (Agnew et al. 1966; Mendels and Hawkins 1967; Schmidt and Kaelbling 1971). Most sleep disorders centers, however, are unwilling to require three or even two nights of diagnostic polysomnography because of the high cost to the patient. One or two attempts have been made to investigate this problem. Although no consensus has been reached, most hypnotic efficacy protocols utilize three consecutive nights of recording to establish basal sleep parameters. It has been claimed that the first night effect is absent or minimal in insomniacs and elderly subjects (Webb and Campbell 1979). On the other hand, Scharf et al. (1975) feel that there will be a "first night effect" even when insomniacs return to the sleep laboratory after sleeping at home for several nights.

A final issue is the effect of the laboratory itself upon objective sleep parameters in chronic insomnia. Several studies suggest that home versus laboratory recordings are comparable (Globus et al. 1974; Coates et al. 1979). New technology involving ambulatory monitors may some day make sleep recordings in the home environment routine.

## 7. Objective Daytime Sleepiness in Chronic Insomnia

Sleep and wakefulness are complementary phases in the daily cycle of human existence. The most obvious relationship between the two phases other than their sequential occurrence in each succeeding 24-hour day is the effect of sleep reduction at night on the following day's level of alertness. We have all experienced sleepiness in our daily lives, most commonly when we must stay awake far beyond our usual bedtime and must get out of bed in the morning for work, travel, or some specific occasion that demands our presence. On such days, most of us have experienced bouts of extreme sleepiness or drowsiness. We may also call these feelings fatigue, tiredness, weariness, and so forth; but they are different from physical tiredness brought about by hard and prolonged physical labor. This distinction is underscored by the fact that nearly everyone will begin to feel sleepy sooner or later in the late evening, and sleepiness at this time bears no obvious relationship to the physical activities of the previous day. It is simply that the brain (or its circadian clock) has decided that it is time to go to bed, and the feeling or state of increasing sleepiness motivates the appropriate behavior.

In recent years, the relationship between nighttime sleep and daytime sleepiness has been studied in some detail (Carskadon 1982; Carskadon and Dement 1979, 1981a; Carskadon et al. 1980a, 1980b; Dement and Carskadon 1981). Although one cannot exist without the other, they are usually considered as entirely separate entities.

A problem remains regarding complaining patients whose sleep parameters seem to be normal. Do they need more sleep, and if so, will the lack of "adequate" sleep be reflected in an associated daytime drowsiness? In truth, insomnia should be regarded as a 24-hour problem. Yet, any approach to evaluating daytime parameters in insomnia has many of the same difficulties described with regard to assessing nocturnal disturbance, such as specifying standard conditions. Daytime sleepiness can be measured and even quantified subjectively, and as a result of the development of the multiple sleep latency test (MSLT) in recent years, it can be measured and quantified objectively (Richardson et al. 1978). Studies of objective or physiological daytime sleepiness in normal volunteers have shown conclusively that sleep at night and wakefulness in the daytime are interacting phases of the daily cycle. Thus daytime sleepiness increases more or less linearly as nocturnal sleep is reduced in experimental subjects (Carskadon and Dement 1982). At the present time, there has been no experimental attempt to duplicate in normal subjects the type of reduction in total sleep time seen in at least some insomniacs; namely, numerous, relatively brief arousals. Presumably, such an approach would increase daytime sleepiness.

Highly relevant to chronic insomnia are the studies of Carskadon and her colleagues in which they measure daytime sleepiness (MSLT) before, during, and after a week of partial sleep deprivation (Carskadon and Dement 1981 a). There is no question from these results (Fig. 5) that a relatively small reduction of sleep produces a substantial and highly significant increase in daytime sleepiness. It is appropriate, therefore, to ask the question, are chronic insomniacs sleepy in the daytime?

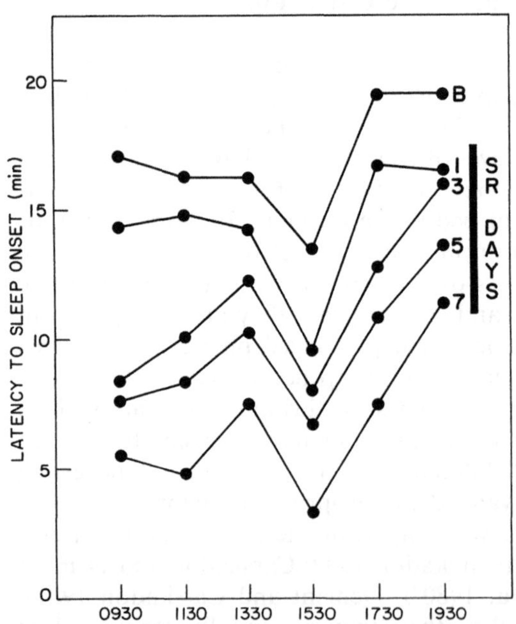


**Fig. 5.** Average daily sleep latency test scores are shown for 10 young adult subjects whose nocturnal sleep was restricted to 5 h on seven consecutive nights. B = baseline sleep tendency curve averaged from 3 nights when subjects slept approximately 9 h. Days 1, 3, 5 and 7 represent days during the sleep restriction condition

This question has recently been addressed by Seidel and Dement (1982) who have accumulated MSLT data on 75 chronic insomniacs. Age-matched control data are sparse; however, the surprising fact is that although some insomniacs are very sleepy and some are moderately sleepy, a substantial number are not sleepy at all in the daytime. The correlation with amount of sleep at night is poor. In other words, the habitual amount of sleep at night, insofar as it was characterized in these studies, did not predict the degree of daytime sleepiness.

What about insomniacs who appear to be fully alert in the daytime? Many investigators have a tendency, when considering insomnia, to regard alertness and anxiety as synonymous. In many patients, however, the presence of unusual anxiety can be satisfactorily ruled out by clinical interview, mood-related questionnaires, and psychophysiological measures. When anxiety is not an impediment to falling asleep during the MSLT, the only feasible ways to account for the chronic insomniac who is fully alert in the daytime are (a) to assume that these subjects fit the definition of "pseudo-insomniacs", subjects who are getting all the sleep they need and somehow feel they should be getting more, or for whom a concern about sleep is a neurotic symptom, or (b) to assume that there are some patients who lack the normal response to sleep reduction. An obvious test of the latter possibility would be to deprive such patients of sleep.

## 8. Longitudinal Aspects of Insomnia

Longitudinal data on insomnia are sparse. We know almost nothing about the natural history of various types of insomnia problems. For example, we do not know the spontaneous remission rate. Unfortunately, the so-called "long-term" (4–5 weeks) drug studies have rarely employed placebo control groups. We have recently carried out a study in which chronic insomniacs were maintained on placebo capsules for six consecutive weeks (Mitler et al., in press). These results show a gradual, consistent, week by week increase in total sleep time (Fig. 6).

What about transient insomnia? It should be possible to describe the entire longitudinal course of transient insomnia. We would expect that some sort of situational event in the life of a normal sleeper (with normal daytime alertness) would be associated with an obvious decrease in total sleep time and an increase in number of nocturnal arousals. Because the time frame of transient insomnia is sufficiently brief, we should be able to document both the change in nighttime sleep and a decrease in daytime alertness. It is conceivable that if the transient insomnia is associated with severe anxiety there would not be a measurable change in daytime alertness on MSLT. The patient should certainly complain of fatigue, weariness, and loss of energy.

In view of the great heterogeneity of chronic insomnia, it is not easy to develop a conceptual model of the natural history. It seems reasonable, as a first approximation, to assume that the premorbid condition was associated with "normal" sleep and reasonable daytime alertness. Unfortunately, adequate normative data on daytime sleepiness in middle-aged adults are lacking. Anecdotally, many adults appear to exploit the trade-off between amount of nocturnal sleep and level of daytime alertness. They give up an hour or two of sleep and pay for their

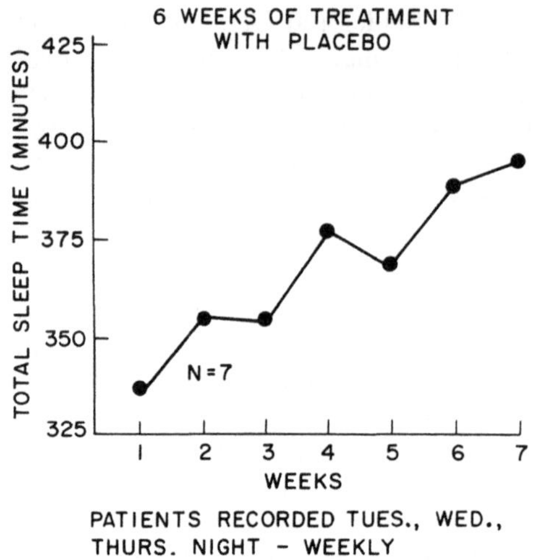


**Fig. 6.** Total sleep time was seen to increase progressively in seven chronic insomniacs administered placebo every night for six weeks (week 1 was without any pill). Sleep was recorded Tuesday, Wednesday and Thursday of each week

"gain" of wake time by enduring a certain degree of chronic sleepiness in the daytime. This sleepiness is generally a minimal problem unless the daytime occupation is completely sedentary. A well-studied benchmark for the simultaneous specification of nocturnal sleep and daytime alertness is the early adolescent, who has very good sleep – long and continuous – associated with optimal daytime alertness. It would be interesting to know if people at successively older ages can achieve this degree of optimal sleep-wake function (which may also involve synchrony of scheduled sleep times with the circadian sleep phase). Can we assume that as insomnia develops and as sleep becomes more and more inadequate, there will be a point at which daytime fatigue, sleepiness, and general dysphoria motivate concerted attempts to achieve more sleep at night, and failing this, chronic symptoms of insomnia develop? Although this model has face validity, it certainly does not fit all chronic insomniacs.

## 9. What Are the Diagnoses (Causes?) of Insomnia?

### 9.1 Overview

Insomnia is a symptom. We would like to assume that sleep is always objectively disturbed in patients who complain of insomnia, but we cannot. Nevertheless, we must ask what causes the complaint. We also hope that when insomnia and objective sleep disturbance co-exist, there is a single cause of both.

Certain aspects of the complaint will point to a specific diagnosis. Usually, however, a diagnostic evaluation of the patient with insomnia must go beyond interview and conventional physical examination. The next step is a comprehensive evaluation of physiological functions during sleep, a test called *clinical polysomnography* (Mitler and Dement 1981).

During the first formal meeting of the Association of Sleep Disorders Centers (ASDC) in 1976, a committee was appointed to organize and standardize a diagnostic system for the sleep and arousal disorders, one that would include all conditions encountered clinically. The resulting document was published as the *Diagnostic Classification of Sleep and Arousal Disorders* in Volume 2 (1) of *Sleep* (ASDC 1979). The system gives clear criteria that can be used by sleep disorders specialists and practicing physicians. It would be inappropriate to give a detailed description of every individual diagnosis of insomnia in the present paper; the original text should be consulted for details. We will briefly describe some of the highlights of this nosology to give a clear flavor of the heterogeneity of insomnia conditions. Finally, it is likely that additional entities are yet to be described.

Several overall categories can be mentioned. One category includes the persistent sleep/wake schedule disorders. Another includes those disorders in which chronic pathophysiology produces multiple arousals. The best examples of this second category are sleep apnea, in which each apneic episode is terminated by an arousal; nocturnal myoclonus, in which the periodic leg movement induces periodic arousal; gastroesophageal reflux, in which acid contents in the distal esophagus have an arousing effect; and conditions associated with nocturnal pain that repeatedly interrupts sleep. A third category includes specific sleep disorder diagnoses for which causality of an objective sleep disturbance is difficult to specify. Two examples are insomnia associated with character and personality disorder and mild depression; and persistent psychophysiological insomnia.

## 9.2 Transient Insomnias

There are two specific primary causes of transient insomnia. The first is a sleep/awake schedule disorder in which either the scheduled sleep hours are shifted, or in which the individual travels rapidly to another time zone and his internal sleep phase thereby becomes out of phase with the scheduled bedtime hours. In either case, sleep is disturbed and there is increased daytime sleepiness. The other primary cause of transient insomnia is the impact of a disturbing situation upon sleep, such as emotional trauma, noise, stimulation, grief, anxiety, and so forth. It has been estimated that jet lag or shift work affect more than 100,000,000 Americans annually, and that transient situational insomnia affects an equal number. In both types of transient insomnia, it is likely that therapeutic intervention would be helpful.

There are instances where severe stress (a typical example might involve loss of job) could conceivably go on for quite a long time. There is no evidence whatsoever that stress applied over several weeks will be associated with insomnia that remains uniform. It seems more reasonable, given what we know about normal sleep, to expect fluctuating insomnia as sleepiness builds up and is then relieved and so on. At any rate, one could well understand a person going through a period of several weeks of stress during which time they would have more or less difficulty sleeping on any given night. This would be diagnosed as transient situational insomnia. If the environmental stress and the insomnia continued, at some arbitrary point it would be called chronic. There is no widely accepted definition of chronicity.

### 9.3 Psychophysiological Insomnia

Persistent psychophysiological insomnia may be due to a cyclic process beginning with transient insomnia, in which the place of sleep or the attempt to sleep becomes associated with frustration and arousal, thereby increasing the sleep loss. Cognitive and environmental stimuli lead to a conditioned arousal response at sleep onset. An important aspect of the diagnosis is to rule out associated psychiatric problems. In older individuals, multiple arousals through the night are usually more common than prolonged sleep latency.

### 9.4 Psychiatric Insomnia

Psychiatric disturbances are often associated with a complaint of insomnia. Personality disorders may lead to hypochondriacal complaints of poor sleep and to actual poor sleep. Unipolar affective disorder commonly includes repeated awakenings and early-morning wakefulness, reduction of stage 4 sleep, and short REM latency; and this reduction in REM latency may be more significant among the elderly (Kupfer 1976). Mania appears to be accompanied by reduced total sleep time, but sleep studies of this disorder are difficult. Kales et al. (1976) present strong arguments for a psychological process underlying the complaint of insomnia. MMPI profiles of 85% of their 128 insomniacs were in the pathological range on one or more of the eight clinical scales. Other investigators have not obtained such a high percentage. Any patient who complains of insomnia and has an associated psychiatric diagnosis would fit here even if another insomnia diagnosis were present, e.g. nocturnal myoclonus.

### 9.5 Insomnia Associated with Use of Drugs or Alcohol

Prolonged use of drugs or alcohol frequently affects sleep adversely. Tolerance to or withdrawal from a wide variety of sedative/hypnotics and other CNS depressants can produce insomnia. Sustained use of stimulants may be implicated. Drugs used to treat non-sleep disorders in the aged may secondarily induce insomnia. Such drugs include theophylline and isoproterenol used to reverse bronchospasm, diphenylhydantoin, and L-DOPA. Tricyclic antidepressants may exacerbate nocturnal myoclonus (Guilleminault et al. 1976b), and their withdrawal may induce rebound REM sleep and nightmares. The use of diuretics will increase nocturia and disrupt sleep. Alcohol, though generally considered soporific, may also produce fragmented sleep after excessive use or upon withdrawal.

### 9.6 Sleep-induced Ventilatory Impairment

Although often associated with excessive daytime somnolence, sleep-induced ventilatory impairment may present as insomnia. The type of apnea associated with the complaint of insomnia is often predominantly central (Guilleminault et al.

1973, 1976a). In predominantly central sleep apnea, snoring may be present, but other complaints seen in upper airway sleep apnea are usually not prominent. The most typical description of the sleep disturbance is a short sleep latency with multiple nocturnal arousals. The older the insomniac, the more likely sleep apnea is to be the cause (Coleman et al. 1981).

### 9.7 Periodic Leg Movement During Sleep (Sleep-related Myoclonus)

First described by Symonds in 1953 as nocturnal myoclonus, periodic leg movement consists of repetitive movements of the lower extremities during sleep, including rapid partial flexion of the foot at the ankle, extension of the big toe, and partial flexion at the knee and hip (Guilleminault et al. 1975; Lugaresi et al. 1970). These movements last several seconds and there is complete relaxation until the next movement, which invariably occurs approximately 25–30 s later. The periodicity and stereotypy are the most distinguishing features of the movements. The actual intensity of the movements can range from a nearly invisible contraction of the anterior tibialis muscle to a violent movement of both lower extremities. When the movements are vigorous and continual over long periods of time, their ability to cause interrupted sleep and insomnia is obvious. Nocturnal myoclonus has, however, been described in persons who do not have a sleep-awake complaint (Kales et al. 1982). In such cases, the frequency and intensity of movements is typically minimal. Coleman et al. (1982a) reported 53 cases in which periodic leg movements during sleep were almost equally associated with the complaint of insomnia and the complaint of excessive daytime sleepiness. A related disorder, restless legs syndrome (Ekbom 1960), is also a cause of insomnia and can be extremely severe.

### 9.8 Persistent Disorders of the Sleep-Wake Schedule

The explicit notion that sleep disorders diagnoses can be made in the area of biological rhythms is quite recent, although it has long been known that schedule changes, shift work, and transmeridian travel can lead to sleep disturbance. There are several persistent disorders in this category. One of the most important, Delayed Sleep Phase Syndrome, has recently been successfully treated by a new technique called "chronotherapy" (Czeisler et al. 1981). This approach utilizes schedule manipulations based upon knowledge about the phase response functions of circadian oscillators.

## 10. What is the Relative Prevalence of Specific Disorders of Insomnia?

More than 5,000 patient records from eleven fully accredited sleep disorders centers accumulated over a two-year period were analyzed in a cooperative study (Coleman et al. 1982b). The major analysis was done on 4,698 cases who were evaluated using all-night clinical polysomnography (NPSG), the basic diagnostic test in sleep-wake disorders medicine. All patients were diagnosed according to the Association of Sleep Disorders Center Classification System. The diagnostic process is based upon analysis of the clinical findings and epoch-by-epoch scoring of the polysomnogram. The emphasis is placed upon diagnosing the patient's current sleep-wake condition. Multiple diagnoses were ranked in order of their importance in explaining the patient's current sleep-wake functioning.

Excluding cases evaluated for nocturnal penile tumescence and patients complaining of excessive daytime sleepiness, Table 1 shows that the most prevalent diagnosis for a Disorder of Initiating or Maintaining Sleep (DIMS) was DIMS associated with psychiatric disorders (35%). This category refers to patients with diagnosable psychiatric disorders as described in DSM-II and currently, DSM-III. Among this large group, approximately half of the patients had a major affective disorder and half had personality disorders, while fewer than 5% had major psychoses. Psychophysiological DIMS (15%) was the second most frequent insomnia diagnosis, followed by drug and alcohol dependency (12.4%), and sleep-related myoclonus and restless legs syndrome (12.2%). Nearly 9% of patients presenting with complaints of insomnia had no significant sleep pathology. Sleep apnea syndromes accounted for 6.2% of DIMS. There can be no question that sleep apnea is a cause of the complaint of insomnia – not the most common, but by no means the most rare.

Only 115 patients (2.9%) were diagnosed within the category of Disorders of the Sleep-Wake Schedule (DSWS). The majority of these disorders have been described recently. Patients in this category typically present with complaints of insomnia, although some patients will complain of excessive sleepiness or specifically indicate a sleep-wake schedule disturbance. Diagnosis of many of these patients was based upon 24-hour ambulatory temperature studies instead of nocturnal polysomnograms. Diaries of sleep-wake schedules together with these monitors usually give sufficient evidence to confirm the clinical impression of a schedule disorder. Because many clinics did not have appropriate diagnostic equipment and the conditions have been described only recently, this category is probably underrepresented.

Among the Sleep-wake Schedule Disorders, Delayed Sleep-Phase Syndrome was the most frequent diagnosis. In this disorder, the patient's 24-hour tempera-

**Table 1.** ASDC case series breakdown of DIMS

| Diagnostic category | *N* | % DIMS | % Range/ Center | % total |
|---|---|---|---|---|
| Psychiatric disorders | 424 | 34.9 | 3.9–66.8 | 10.9 |
| Psychophysiological | 186 | 15.3 | 1.0–32.9 | 4.8 |
| Drug and alcohol dependency | 151 | 12.4 | 2.9–25.2 | 3.9 |
| Sleep related myoclonus and RLS [a] | 148 | 12.2 | 2.8–26.3 | 3.8 |
| No insomnia abnormality | 112 | 9.2 | 0.0–28.7 | 2.9 |
| Sleep apnea syndromes | 75 | 6.2 | 0.0–18.4 | 1.9 |
| Other insomnia conditions | 68 | 5.6 | 0.0–12.6 | 1.7 |
| Medical, toxic and environmental | 46 | 3.8 | 0.0–12.6 | 1.2 |
| Childhood-onset insomnia | 4 | 0.3 | 0.0– 1.6 | 0.1 |
| Totals | 1214 | 99.9 | | 31.2 |

[a] RLS indicates restless legs syndrome

ture rhythm is usually delayed three or more hours relative to the pattern seen in individuals with conventional sleeping times. As a result, these patients have severe objective sleep-onset insomnia.

### Comment

The major message of this cooperative study is that a fully developed clinical specialty of the diagnosis and treatment of sleep disorders exists. The formulation of precise definitions and clinical descriptions of specific disorders is a crucial developmental landmark.

The cooperative case series study represents the largest analysis of sleep-wake disorders to date utilizing polysomnographic diagnosis and a common nosology. A second compilation is in progress, but the results are essentially the same. The proportions of specific diagnoses *within* the complaint categories may be essentially the same as in the general population; the major distincton is that sleep disorders centers do not evaluate patients with brief insomnia. Nevertheless, we cannot assume that this case series is a representative sample of patients with persistent insomnia that will be encountered by physicans until sleep disorders center diagnostic evaluations are done in this patient group. It seems reasonable, however, that this series can provide reasonable expectations for medical practice.

## 11. How Should We Regard Disturbed Sleep in Noncomplaining Subjects?

We asked the question earlier: can we call an individual who has severe sleep disturbance and no complaint an insomniac? The answer is essentially a matter of definition. From a common sense point of view, we would certainly hesitate to deny heart disease in a man with blocked coronary arteries and ECG changes just because he had no chest pain. In the same way, there are now plentiful reports of individuals, particularly older individuals, who may have hundreds of arousals during sleep, but who do not complain either of disturbed sleep or daytime sleepiness. By analogy, we could certainly classify such individuals under the rubric of insomnia, although disturbed sleep *per se* is not as clearly a pathology as blocked coronary arteries. The solution to this dilemma depends upon what we consider the most important factor in insomnia: complaining about sleep or having an objective disturbance. When people complain bitterly of insomnia, we tend to take it seriously regardless of objective sleep parameters. By the same token, if there is no complaint at all, sleep has to be impressively disturbed to be of concern. All of this goes to show that the problem of insomnia is exceedingly complicated.

In addition to all the other factors involved in insomnia, age is one of the most important. Numerous surveys show that insomnia is more prevalent in older populations (Miles and Dement 1980; Dement et al. 1982a). Furthermore, the tendency for sleep to be disturbed and fragmented increases markedly with age, independent of complaint. We cannot at present be sure what represents "normal" aging and what is an age-related increase in pathology.

**Table 2.** Apneas during sleep in noncomplaining healthy volunteers

| | Middle aged | Elderly |
|---|---|---|
| *N* | 24 (12 M 12 F) | 40 (18 M 22 F) |
| Mean age: | 49.9 | 73.8 |
| Age range: | 48–60 | 62–86 |
| Mean respiration disturbances/night: | 4.7 | 50.0 |
| Range respiration disturbances/night: | 0–12 | 0–216 |
| Number with RDI > 5 | 0 | 15 |

Respiration disturbance = apnea or hypopnea
Hypopnea = 50% reduction of breathing > 10 s, terminating in arousal
Apnea = Respiratory pause > 10 s
RDI = Respiration disturbance index (number of respiration disturbances/hour of sleep)

Sleep apnea is ofen related to disturbed sleep in noncomplainers. Studies of healthy asymptomatic elderly subjects have yielded the most dramatic and unexpected results. For example, Carskadon and Dement (1981 b) selected elderly volunteers on the basis of having no complaint about their sleep and no serious health problem. These volunteers were felt to be the group most likely to have good (undisturbed) sleep and normal respiration during sleep. Table 2 shows the results from 40 elderly subjects compared to 24 middle-aged subjects.

The large difference in mean number of respiratory disturbances between the two groups is highly significant. Recalling that each apneic pause is terminated by an arousal, we may conclude that 37.5% of the elderly subjects experience five or more interruptions of their sleep per hour, and 30% had ten or more interruptions per hour. These findings suggest that age-related respiratory impairment may account for a great deal of the fragmentation in elderly subjects reported by many investigators (Miles and Dement 1980). Similar data have been reported by Krieger et al. (1981), Smythe et al. (1981), McGinty et al. (1981), and Ancoli-Israel et al. (1981).

In summary, there are many individuals who show hundreds of arousals per night. Some of these individuals feel that there sleep is normal – they have no complaint (Carskadon et al. 1982a). What should take precedence, objective sleep disturbance or subjective perception of sleep disturbance? At the present time, it is the complaint only which motivates patients to seek treatment. It is possible to visualize a future time when noncomplaining individuals are routinely screened and when objective sleep disturbance might be treated in the absence of a complaint.

## 12. What Are the Proper Criteria of Hypnotic Efficacy?

Sleeping pills are generally defined as compounds that induce and maintain sleep. There is a rather large number of compounds for which this claim has been made – alcohol, antihistamines, phenothiazines, tricyclic antidepressants, benzodiazepines, barbiturates, antihypertensives, amino acids, vitamins, and certain foods such as milk, plus nonchemical agents such as heat, exercise, relaxation, and so forth. The single family of compounds most widely used worldwide at the present time to induce sedation and/or drowsiness and/or sleep is the benzodiazepines. The main reason for this pre-eminence is their high degree of safety.

There has been a tendency in past years for investigators to confuse two goals of hypnotic drug evaluation. The first goal is to answer the question, does the compound reliably induce and maintain sleep? The second goal is to determine if the compound effectively treats some individual patient or group of patients. The first question is typically answered by administering the compound to a small group of chronic insomniacs who have a severe objective sleep disturbance. From large amounts of sleep laboratory data on chronic insomniacs, we know that such a group is highly unrepresentative. It is not uncommon to screen as many as 50 chronic insomnia patients to find one who meets such objective sleep parameter criteria (Dement et al. 1978). One wonders why this question is not answered in a less heroic manner, utilizing middle-aged to elderly subjects with or without insomnia, but with sufficient objective sleep disturbance to show a clear change.

Whereas approaches to the first goal can be made easier and simpler, approaches to the second goal must allow for great complexity. Patients should be grouped by diagnosis as homogeneously as possible, and the benefit desired by the patient and/or the physician should be clearly specified. A further point is that sleeping pills are intended to provide symptomatic relief, not specific treatment. Symptomatic improvement or relief of insomnia means that the perceived sleep disturbance and its perceived daytime consequences are decreased or entirely abolished. Finally, it is conceivable that the benefit the patient is seeking is not in his best interest. Thus, the physician may have a different therapeutic goal based on his expert evaluation of the patient and his knowledge about sleep disorders.

## 12.1 Nocturnal Criteria of Hypnotic Efficacy

Many assumptions have been made about the process underlying symptomatic relief of insomnia. In particular, it is assumed that there is a parallel improvement in objective sleep parameters. The effect of sleeping pills on the symptoms of insomnia in patients whose sleep parameters show little room for improvement (Carskadon et al. 1976) has never been systematically studied; however, one pilot study showed minimal or no increase in sleep time with medication when basal sleep times were near seven hours (Hoddes et al. 1972). As noted above, regardless of what we measure to establish efficacy, the ultimate goal in clinical practice is to be able to say that a particular sleeping pill at a particular dose is effective in relieving the symptoms of insomnia in a particular patient. If symptomatic relief is not obtained for that patient, the medication is not effective, regardless of whether his sleep parameters have changed or whether efficacy has been established in previous scientific studies.

Studies in the sleep laboratory deal with changes in objective sleep parameters. Observations are carried out on relatively small numbers of subjects with the attendant difficulty in generalizing. An effective hypnotic should, in a sleep laboratory situation, shorten or reduce the sleep latency, increase the total amount of sleep, and reduce the amount of nocturnal wakefulness. All benzodiazepines appear to be able objectively to induce and maintain sleep if an adequate dose is administered. The issue which has never been addressed is what are the quantitative criteria of efficacy – how large should the changes in sleep be for a particular dose of the drug to be deemed effective? This is really a "dose-ranging" problem, however, and if a given dose of a compound statistically significantly increases sleep time by a small amount, one can increase the dose to increase the size of the effect. Nonetheless, some investigators declare a statistically significant change of as little as 10 minutes in a sleep parameter over the entire night a demonstration of efficacy. Perhaps a reasonable standard would be to expect a change of at least 60 minutes, which could be a combination of reduced sleep latency, reduced intra-sleep wakefulness, and/or increased length of the sleep period. Another possibility might be to ask the patient how much sleep he considers normal and use this amount as the criterion.

Because of the emphasis on objective sleep parameters, subjective parameters are often overlooked. What does it mean if objective parameters are improved but the patient does not perceive an improvement? To some extent, this may reflect the inherent difficulty with subjective assessment of sleep. It is unlikely, however, that patients will use medications they feel are ineffective.

## 12.2 Daytime Criteria of Hypnotic Efficacy

Our view at the Stanford University Sleep Center is that the entire 24-hour day must be assessed when we are evaluating the efficacy of sleeping pills. With this view in mind, we advance the modest proposition that if sleep is improved at night, there ought to be a corresponding improvement in daytime function. This proposition has been substantiated in normal volunteers utilizing levels of alertness as the measure of daytime function and non-drug methods of improving sleep (Dement and Carskadon 1981; Carskadon and Dement 1982). However daytime function is assessed, it ought to include some objective measures, because it has been shown that daytime performance testing can be seriously impaired even though the patient insists that his function is improved (IOM 1979; Linnoila et al. 1980).

A focus on daytime changes also presents the advantage that efficacy criteria will not depend solely on exceeding some arbitrary value in nocturnal sleep parameters. Indeed, from a quantitative point of view, the typically reported nocturnal changes seem almost irrelevant. Finally, the insomniac who does not care about feeling better in the daytime may be the exception rather than the rule. At any rate, it seems reasonable to ask if effectively inducing and maintaining sleep also improves, or at least does not worsen, daytime alertness. The probable reason that this issue has been so widely ignored has been the lack of reliable methods for measuring daytime sleepiness. This obstacle has been overcome. Furthermore, copious information on the pharmacokinetics of benzodiazepines has been accumulated, which will allow us to interpret the daytime effects of nighttime hypnotics (Breimer 1979; Greenblatt et al. 1981).

Many investigators (Church and Johnson 1979; Hindmarch and Clyde 1980; Johnson and Chernik 1982; Linnoila et al. 1980; Nicholson and Stone 1980; Oswald et al. 1979; Roth et al. 1980, 1981; Spinweber and Johnson 1982) have utilized performance testing to assess daytime function. In this approach, the detection of impairment is interpreted as indicating daytime carryover of nocturnal sedative effects. At Stanford, we have utilized the direct measurement of daytime sleepiness/alertness levels before, during, and after treatment with benzodiazepines. Daytime sleepiness as a basal attribute of chronic insomnia was briefly considered earlier in this paper.

We define sleepiness operationally as the tendency to fall asleep. A precise measure of the tendency to fall asleep is possible using standard sleep laboratory techniques. The measure, called the Multiple Sleep Latency Test (MSLT), simply involves determining the time it takes to fall asleep five or six times across a single day. Precise details of the procedure are described in numerous publications (cf. Carskadon 1982; Mitler 1982).

The MSLT has been used to measure physiological sleep tendency in a number of conditions (Carskadon and Dement 1979; Carskadon and Dement 1981 a; Carskadon et al. 1980 a, 1980 b; Dement et al. 1978 b; Richardson et al. 1978). We have found that the single group with the most consistent pattern of alertness across the day is the 10- to 12-year-old prepubescent adolescent. These children sleep through the night for more than nine hours; when they awake, they are alert and energetic all day with a physiological sleep tendency that is per-

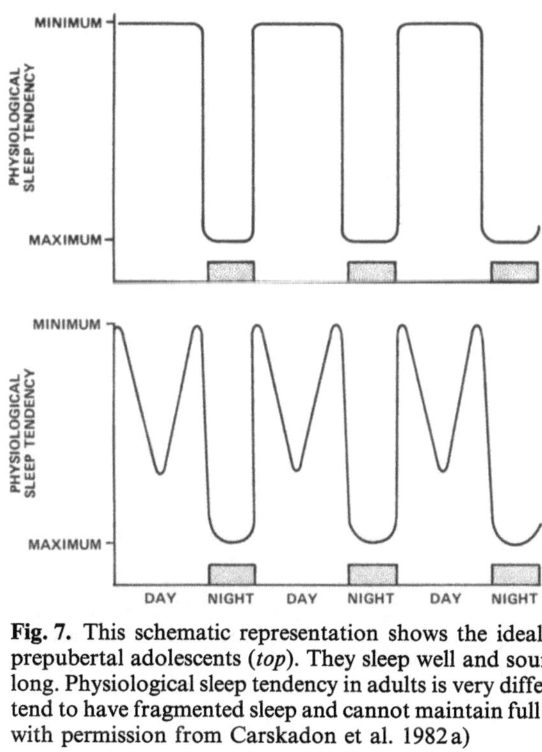


**Fig. 7.** This schematic representation shows the ideal synchrony of sleep and wakefulness in prepubertal adolescents (*top*). They sleep well and soundly at night and are wide awake all day long. Physiological sleep tendency in adults is very different from children (*bottom*). Older adults tend to have fragmented sleep and cannot maintain full alertness throughout the day. (Reprinted with permission from Carskadon et al. 1982 a)

sistently at or near zero. In contrast, older persons consistently show a greater degree of physiological sleep tendency in the daytime (Carskadon et al. 1980b). In the elderly, sleep at night is typically disturbed, and there is a clear tendency for increased physiological sleepiness during the day.

The MSLT has received nearly unanimous clinical application in sleep disorders centers across the country (Mitler 1982). Its primary use to date has been in the daytime evaluation of patients suspected to have narcolepsy or sleep apnea. Preliminary results of its use to evaluate basal sleepiness in patients with chronic insomnia have also been reported (Seidel and Dement 1982; Dement et al. 1982b). Fig. 7 shows the idealized optimal sleepiness/alertness pattern that generally characterizes 10- to 12-year-olds together with the typical pattern of sleepiness/alertness in older persons, as well as samples of patients with narcolepsy and sleep apnea.

The MSLT is remarkably sensitive to changes in the amount of sleep at night. Daytime latencies to sleep onset decline (sleep tendency increases) with incremental reductions of nocturnal sleep, or lengthen with incremental increases (Carskadon and Dement 1982).

## 12.3 Changes in Daytime Alertness After Bedtime Administration of Hypnotics: Flurazepam and Triazolam in Normal Subjects

Since the principle action of sedative-hypnotic drugs is "to produce drowsiness" (Harvey 1980), the direct assessment of this quality in the daytime should be of particular value in determining whether a nocturnal medication is continuing to act. Since at least one purpose of improving sleep at night is to improve alertness in the daytime, a change in daytime alertness in either direction would be clinically significant. We describe here the results of studies in which the daytime effects of the bedtime administration of a long-acting benzodiazepine (flurazepam) were compared with the daytime effects of a short-acting benzodiazepine (triazolam). The studies involved 24-hour measurement in scheduled bed periods with MSLT and performance testing all through the following day. Only the MSLT data will be described in this paper.

In the first study, eleven healthy noncomplaining adult subjects were evaluated on a 24-hour basis before and during treatment with sleeping pills in order

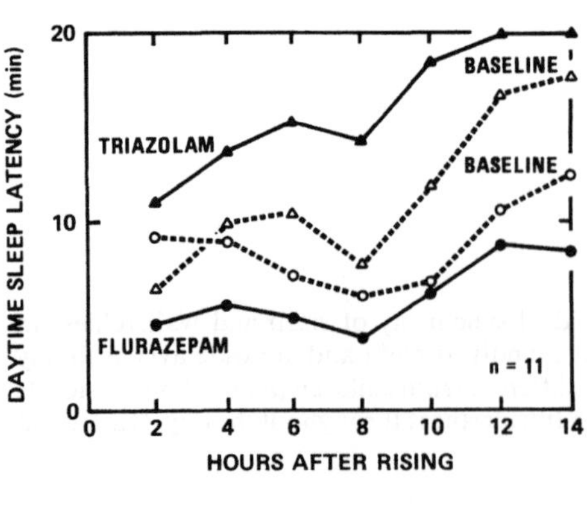


**Fig. 8.** Effects of 0.5 mg triazolam and 30 mg flurazepam on MSLT profiles of normal sleepers. Each point is the mean of 2 days testing with 5 (flurazepam group) or 6 (triazolam group) subjects. Baseline sleepiness for the flurazepam group was lower, but the effects of treatments are strikingly opposite. (Reprinted with permission from Dement et al. 1982b)

to demonstrate drug effects uncomplicated by insomnia. In a parallel groups design, subjects took no medication for the first three nights, then received either 0.5 mg triazolam or 30 mg flurazepam 30 min before lights out for the next seven nights. Baseline daytime testing occurred after nights 2 and 3, and testing during the treatment period was done after the third and seventh nights of medicated sleep.

The two baseline days were averaged within groups, as were the two days of testing during treatment. Although the baselines did not match, the direction of the medication effects were clearly opposite.The MSLT results are shown in Fig. 8. These changes in daytime sleepiness appeared to occur without substantial changes in the amount of sleep at night. Transient arousals were not assessed. Daytime alertness was increased with triazolam and decreased with flurazepam.

## 12.4 Changes in Daytime Alertness after Bedtime Administration of Hypnotics: Flurazepam and Triazolam in Chronic Insomniacs

To investigate further the differential effect of triazolam and flurazepam on daytime drowsiness, a multi-center cooperative study was undertaken involving Sleep Disorders Centers at Stanford University, Baylor University, Henry Ford Hospital, and New York University at Stonybrook, using a counterbalanced crossover design; placebo, 7 days of treatment one, 2 weeks of placebo/washout, then finally 7 days of treatment two. Again, the treatments were 30 mg flurazepam and 0.5 mg triazolam at bedtime. The subjects were patients with chronic insomnia, defined as a persistent complaint of poor nocturnal sleep plus a complaint about daytime functioning. The MSLT was administered on the days after laboratory nights 2 and 3 on both baselines, and after treatment nights 6 and 7 for both treatment periods.

The two baseline MSLT's were essentially identical for each subject in this population, which suggests that in the absence of treatment or other manipulation of nocturnal sleep, daytime sleepiness is a reasonable stable characteristic.

Details of the entire study are published elsewhere (Bliwise et al. 1983). We present here some of the MSLT data on five patients studied at Stanford. Average sleep latency profiles are presented in Fig. 9. The five patients exhibited increased daytime drowsiness after 7 days of flurazepam, and substantially less drowsiness

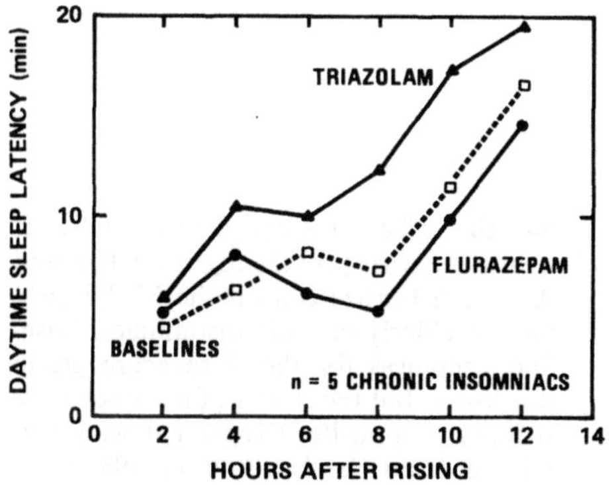


**Fig. 9.** Effect of 1 week of nightly treatment with 0.5 mg triazolam or 30 mg flurazepam on the MSLT profiles of 5 chronic insomniacs (every patient received both treatments). Each baseline point is the mean of 4 days; treatment points are the means of 2 days of testing. (Reprinted with permission from Dement et al. 1982b)

after triazolam. The sixth patient completed the triazolam condition, but was forced to drop out due to over-sedation and depression after 3 days in the flurazepam condition.

## 12.5 Changes in Daytime Alertness After Bedtime Administration of Hypnotics: Flurazepam and Triazolam in the Elderly

Very few sleep laboratory studies of hypnotic efficacy in geriatric patients have been published. We have begun a comprehensive program at Stanford University. In one of our first studies (Carskadon et al. 1982b), we evaluated the effects of triazolam 0.25 mg or flurazepam 15 mg in 13 elderly (ages 64–79) insomniacs. Subjects were reasonably healthy, ambulatory, and complained of disturbed sleep. Sleep apnea syndromes were ruled out in this group by nocturnal polysomnogram. Sleep, daytime sleepiness (MSLT), performance, and mood were assessed on 5 consecutive days. Placebo was given on nights 1 and 2; active medications were given on nights 3–5.

Sleep time was increased by approximately one hour in both treatment groups. MSLT showed increased sleepiness with flurazepam and decreased sleepiness with triazolam. The MSLT results are summarized in Fig. 10. Auditory vigilance was impaired with flurazepam and unchanged with triazolam. Other performance tests showed no change. Although both compounds improved sleep

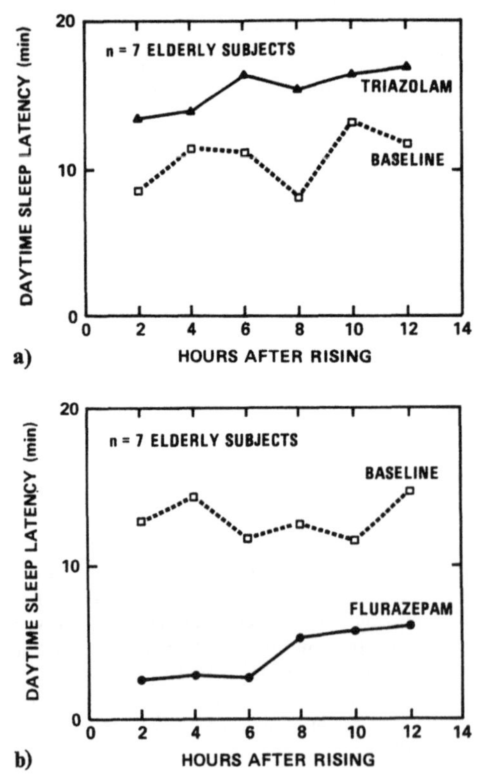


**Fig. 10.** Effect of 3 consecutive nights of treatment with (**a**) 0.25 mg triazolam and (**b**) 15 mg flurazepam on the MSLT profiles of elderly chronic insomniacs. Baseline sleepiness for the flurazepam group was lower, but the effects of treatments are strikingly opposite. (Reprinted with permission from Carskadon et al. 1982b)

at one-half the usual adult doses, there was substantial residual sedation with flurazepam and improved daytime alertness with triazolam. This study suggests that elderly persons may have a greater vulnerability to the daytime carryover of sleeping medication.

In order to determine whether the MSLT changes might be associated with specific changes in nocturnal sleep, we computed correlation coefficients for each subject between daily mean MSLT scores and selected nocturnal sleep parameters. Although none of the individual correlations achieved statistical significance, there was a marked tendency in the triazolam group for high values to be associated with nocturnal measures that would, a priori, seem to be related to daytime sleepiness. Thus, relatively high correlations with MSLT were found for total sleep time, total wake time, minutes and percent of NREM stage 2 sleep, and percentage of NREM stage 1 sleep. In the flurazepam group, on the other hand, correlations tended to cluster around zero.

## 12.6 Comments

We have approached chronic insomnia as a 24-hour problem. We assume that some sort of chronic sleep disturbance underlies the persistent complaint which, in turn, produces feelings in the daytime commonly associated with loss of sleep – namely, drowsiness, weariness, fatigue, loss of initiative, and so forth. Insofar as a bedtime hypnotic corrects the sleep disturbance, it should improve daytime function in some way. The changes we observed in daytime alertness after ingesting benzodiazepines at bedtime were fairly consistent. In general, the short-acting bedtime benzodiazepine was followed by decreased sleep tendency in the daytime. The long-acting benzodiazepine was followed by increased daytime sleepiness.

The simplest interpretation of these results is that the differing effects of longer-acting (i.e., flurazepam) and shorter-acting (i.e., triazolam) benzodiazepines are due to two factors. First, a long half-life implies that the medication will continue to promote sleep in the daytime. The second factor is improved sleep. The improved daytime alertness seen with triazolam may simply be due to getting more sleep at night. In the absence of daytime carryover, the daytime effect of increased nocturnal sleep is unopposed. It also follows that flurazepam subjects might be even sleepier in the daytime if sleep at night were not improved.

What is the meaning of the level of daytime physiological sleep tendency assessed by MSLT? When minimal, we believe that it reflects sustained levels of well-being, zest, or energy throughout the day. When maximal, the daytime sleep tendency reflects intense subjective drowsiness, lethargy, and fatigue; and patients and subjects generally show microsleeps and fall asleep involuntarily, with a corresponding interruption of ongoing behavior or performance. When MSLT profiles indicate moderate sleepiness (i.e., mean sleep latencies between 5 and 10 min), subjects can usually resist falling asleep *except* in sedentary, boring, and other sleep-promoting situations. Accordingly, an increase in physiological sleep tendency simply means that individuals are more likely to fall asleep while driving a car, while listening to a lecture, and so forth. We assume that long-acting benzodiazepines which measurably increase daytime sleep tendencies also increase the probability of falling asleep during routine, nonstimulating behaviors. Finally, improved alertness is desirable in and of itself. Prolonged daytime drowsiness can be miserable. Generally, relief from drowsiness is considered an important effect of "good sleep". Clearly, the zest and ebullience associated with full alertness is a desirable goal for symptomatic treatment.

Finally, the basal alertness of chronic insomniacs could be very important in establishing indications. Improving daytime alertness in someone already fully alert might not be a very meaningful therapeutic goal. Additional daytime sedation of someone already very sleepy might actually be dangerous.

## 13. How Should Hypnotics Be Used in Clinical Practice?

What about the practical, clinical use of benzodiazepine hypnotics? What are the indications for treatment with sleeping pills? What specific benefits do patients desire? Are their expectations appropriate? How do we know if a patient actually benefits from treatment with sleeping pills? Is the patient the best judge of the effect of the treatment? This area was recently reviewed by Roth et al. (1982).

### 13.1 Indications for Use of Hypnotics

Effective use of hypnotics in medical practice has profited from our increasing knowledge about insomnia and a more sophisticated sleep disorders clinic approach to the evaluation of hypnotic efficacy. At the present time, the single most appropriate use of hypnotics is for transient insomnia. This includes situational insomnia due to acute stress, jet lag, and acute shift work change. It should be obvious that in most of these instances, hypnotics will be prescribed prophylactically. Therefore, the physician must know the patient and have confidence in his description or prior transient sleep problems.

Although it is likely that transient insomnia is far more common than chronic insomnia, it has rarely been studied in the sleep laboratory. In addition, transient insomnia is generally not considered to be a serious medical problem. Given that benzodiazepine hypnotics have very high safety and low toxicity, however, are we justified in withholding the opportunity to provide symptomatic relief in situational insomnia, jet lag, and acute shift work change? Tolerance and rebound insomnia should not be problems in treating patients with transient insomnias. Toxicity should not be an issue. On the other hand, absorption, i.e., sleep induction, will be an issue, sleep maintenance will be an issue, and above all, daytime alertness should be an issue. If a patient with transient insomnia is disabled by anxiety in the daytime, a long acting hypnotic might be appropriate. In most cases, however, the promotion of daytime alertness should be a major goal of therapy. At the present time, only one compound, triazolam, has shown improved daytime alertness following bedtime administration.

The chronic use of hypnotics is a more complicated issue. There currently exists little or no information on the efficacy and safety of hypnotics when taken for substantially more than one month. Despite this lack, some speculations can be made. First, it must be recognized that chronic use of hypnotics should not be undertaken until a thorough sleep evaluation (including nocturnal polysomnography) has been done (Zorick et al. 1981). After an evaluation has been performed and cause of the complaint has been documented, a clinical trial with hypnotics might be undertaken with certain patients. Specifically, patients with the diagnoses of persistent psychophysiological insomnia, nocturnal myoclonus, and insomnia associated with selected psychiatric problems may benefit from a trial with hypnotics.

How long should such a clinical trial be continued? What does one month of symptomatic relief mean (assuming we could provide it) compared to a lifetime of having the illness? Taking persistent psychophysiological insomnia as an example, the major issue is whether or not a course of hypnotic therapy could induce a remission. Furthermore, it is known that this condition can be divided into those who are sleepy and those who are alert. Rational clinical guidelines should take these differences into account. The longer the treatment, the greater likelihood of deleterious withdrawal effects (Kales et al. 1978; 1979) or of a tendency to escalate the dose. In addition, the chance of harmful interactions with other drugs increases as a function of increasing length of the period of medication. If a genuine remission of the insomnia does occur, however, then the treatment with hypnotics was beneficial.

The question of exactly when to discontinue treatment is very difficult. Delayed withdrawal effects such as might occur with flurazepam could be more troublesome than immediate withdrawal effects, because the patient might not associate delayed changes with discontinuation of treatment (Mitler et al. in press). Rather, he might erroneously assume that the delayed withdrawal represents his basal condition. Withdrawal might also mask a remission. Remission of chronic insomnia has not been conclusively documented either as the result of treatment or spontaneously. It is also extremely important that the physician keep in mind the documented variability of response to hypnotics (Nicholson et al. 1982). Such variability can include the clinical response to the drug, the development of tolerance, and whether or not there are effects of discontinuation.

It is clear that the physician who elects to treat a patient with hypnotics must evaluate the patient *during* the treatment. Does the patient feel better? Is the initial effect still present? Did the patient actually receive the desired benefit from the medication? At the practical level, the specific dose is very important. A dose that produces a grand total effect on sleep of 10 minutes increase may not be therapeutic. On the other hand, the recommended adult dose may be too high for an individual patient.

## 13.2 Contraindications for Use of Hypnotics

There are several situations in which hypnotics are unequivocally contraindicated. Patients with disturbed sleep associated with sleep apnea should not be given hypnotics (Mendelson et al. 1981; Dolly and Block 1982; Guilleminault et al. in press). Patients who are known to use alcohol excessively should never be given hypnotics. Pregnant women should avoid the use of hypnotics, particularly in the first trimester. Finally, people who are subject to being aroused and required to perform in the middle of the night should avoid hypnotics. All hypnotics that promote sleep increase awakening thresholds and impair the ability to function adequately in the middle of the night.

### 13.3 Special Situations

In certain situations, hypnotics are not clearly contraindicated, but should be prescribed with caution. Hypnotic use in elderly patients always requires careful monitoring (Mattila et al. 1977). In addition to the high prevalence of sleep apnea mentioned above, it takes a great deal longer for elderly patients to metabolize benzodiazepine medications (Greenblatt et al. 1981). Patients with lung, kidney, or liver disease should be carefully monitored for drug toxicity. Patients with drug abuse potential or suicidal risk should be treated with great caution. Finally, drug interactions should be considered. Cimetidine is now widely used and changes the metabolism of benzodiazepines.

## 14. Conclusion – What is the Ideal Hypnotic?

It is clear that we can be much more rational today about issues involving the diagnosis and treatment of insomnia, because we know a great deal more than in the past. We emphasize that the evaluation of insomnia should include attention to the presence of daytime symptoms. We also emphasize that criteria of hypnotic efficacy should include evidence of improvement in daytime symptoms. Generally, the patient should feel more refreshed and alert in the daytime, or the daytime symptoms attributed to sleep disturbance should be ameliorated at the same time that sleep is improved. If daytime symptoms are unchanged, we cannot affirm the efficacy of a particular hypnotic.

In terms of what is already available to practicing physicians, current medications offer a range of possibilities. However, we need more objective information about very prolonged (months to years) efficacy. Because we cannot treat specific causes of insomnia in many cases, we need drugs that will never lose their efficacy and, at the same time, will have no long term deleterious effects. Finally, we need more evidence that hypnotics have no significant deleterious effect on physiology or pathophysiology during sleep.

In conclusion, the ideal hypnotic should improve sleep objectively and subjectively; it should improve daytime function objectively and subjectively; it should sustain its therapeutic effectiveness for the duration needed by a particular patient. The impact of withdrawal should be minimal. Finally, there should be few or no side effects.

## References

Agnew HW, Webb WB, Williams RL (1966) The first night effect: an EEG study of sleep. Psychophysiology 2:263–266

Ancoli-Israel S, Kripke D, Mason W, Messin S (1981) Sleep apnea and nocturnal myoclonus in a senior population. Sleep 4:349–358

Association of Sleep Disorders Centers (1979) Diagnostic classification of sleep and arousal disorders, 1st ed. Prepared by the Sleep Disorders Classification Commitee (HP Roffwarg, Chairman). Sleep 2:1–207

Bliwise D, Seidel W, Karacan I, Mitler M, Roth T, Zorick F, Dement W (1983) Daytime sleepiness as a criterion in hypnotic medication trials: comparison of triazolam and flurazepam. Sleep 6:156–163

Breimer D (1979) Pharmacokinetics and metabolism of various benzodiazepines used as hypnotics. Br J Clin Pharmacol 8:7–13

Březinová V, Catterall J, Douglas N, Calverley P, Flenley D (1982) Night sleep of patients with chronic ventilatory failure and age matched controls: number and duration of the EEG episodes of intervening wakefulness and drowsiness. Sleep 5:123–130

Carskadon MA (1982) The second decade. In: Guilleminault C (ed) Sleeping and waking disorders: Indications and techniques. Addison-Wesley, Menlo Park, CA, pp 99–125

Carskadon M, Brown E, Dement WC (1982a) Sleep fragmentation in the elderly: relationship to daytime sleep tendency. Neurobiol Aging 3:321–327

Carskadon MA, Seidel WF, Greenblatt DJ, Dement WC (1982b) Daytime carryover of triazolam and flurazepam in elderly insomniacs. Sleep 5:361–371

Carskadon M, Dement W (1981) Cumulative effects of sleep restriction on daytime sleepiness. Psychophysiology 18:107–113

Carskadon M, Harvey K, Duke P, Anders T, Litt I, Dement W (1980a) Pubertal changes in daytime sleepiness. Sleep 2:453–460

Carskadon M, van den Hoed J, Dement W (1980b) Sleep and daytime sleepiness in the elderly. J Geriatr Psychiatry 13:135–151

Carskadon M, Dement W (1979) Effects of total sleep loss on sleep tendency. Percept Mot Skills 48:495–506

Carskadon MA, Dement WC, Mitler MM, Guilleminault C, Zarcone VP, Spiegel R (1976) Self-reports versus sleep laboratory findings in 122 drug-free subjects with the complaint of chronic insomnia. Am J Psychiatry 133:1382–1388

Carskadon M, Dement W (1982) Nocturnal determinants of daytime sleepiness. Sleep 5:73–81

Church MW, Johnson LC (1979) Mood and performance of poor sleepers during repeated use of flurazepam. Psychopharmacology (Berlin) 61:309–316

Coates TJ, Rosekind MR, Strossen RJ, Thoresen CE, Kirmil-Gray K (1979) Sleep recordings in the laboratory and home: comparative analysis. Psychophysology 16:339–346

Coleman R, Bliwise D, Sajben N, Boomkamp A, deBruyn L, Dement W (1982a) Daytime sleepiness in patients with periodic movements in sleep. Sleep 5:191–202

Coleman R, Roffwarg H, Kennedy S, Guilleminault C, Cinque J, Cohn M, Karacan I, Kupfer D, Lemmi H, Miles L, Orr W, Phillips E, Roth T, Sassin J, Schmidt H, Weitzman E, Dement W (1982b) Sleep-wake disorders based on a polysomnographic diagnosis: a national cooperative study. JAMA 247:997–1003

Coleman R, Miles L, Guilleminault C, Zarcone V, van den Hoed J, Dement W (1981) Sleep-wake disorders in the elderly: a polysomnographic analysis. J Am Geriatr Soc 29:289–296

Coleman R, Pollak C, Weitzman E (1980) Periodic movements in sleep (nocturnal myoclonus): relation to sleep disorders. Ann Neurol 8:416–421

Czeisler C, Richardson G, Coleman R, Zimmerman J, Moore-Ede M, Dement W, Weitzman E (1981) Chronotherapy: resetting the circadian clocks of patients with delayed sleep phase insomnia. Sleep 4:1–21

Dement W (1982) Sleep disorders and their substrates. Nouv Presse Med. 11:2967–2980

Dement W (in press) Rational basis for the use of sleeping pills. Karger, Basel

Dement W, Carskadon M (1981) An essay on sleepiness. In: Actualités en medecine èxperimentale, en hommage au Professeur P. Passount. Montpellier, France. Euromed, pp 47–71

Dement W, Carskadon M, Mitler M, Phillips R, Zarcone V (1978a) Prolonged use of flurazepam: a sleep laboratory study. Behav Med 5:25–31

Dement W, Carskadon M, Richardson G (1978b) Excessive daytime sleepiness in the sleep apnea syndrome. In: Guilleminault C, Dement W (eds) Sleep Apnea Syndromes. Liss Inc, New York, pp 23–46

Dement WC, Miles LE, Carskadon MA (1982a) "White paper" on sleep and aging. J Am Ger Soc 30(1):25–50

Dement W, Seidel W, Carskadon M (1982b) Daytime alertness, insomnia, and benzodiazepines. Sleep 5:28–45
Dolly F, Block A (1982) Effect of flurazepam on sleep-disordered breathing and nocturnal oxygen desaturation in asymptomatic subjects. JAMA 73:239–243
Ekbom K (1960) Restless legs syndrome. Neurol 10:868–873
Globus G, Phoebus E, Humphries J, Boyd R, Gaffrey D, Gaffrey S (1974) The effect of lorazepam on anxious insomniacs' sleep as recorded in the home environment. J Clin Pharmacol 14:192–201
Greenblatt D, Divoll M, Harmatz J, MacLaughlin D, Shader R (1981) Kinetics and clinical effects of flurazepam in young and old noninsomniacs. Clin Pharmacol Therap 30:475–486
Guilleminault C, Eldridge F, Phillips J, Dement WC (1976a) Two occult causes of insomnia and their therapeutic problems. Arch Gen Psychiatry 33:1241–1245
Guilleminault C, Raynal D, Takahashi S, Carskadon M, Dement W (1976b) Evaluation of short-term and long-term treatment of the narcolepsy syndrome with chlomipramine hydrochloride. Acta Neurol Scand 54:71–87
Guilleminault C, Raynal D, Weitzman E, Dement W (1975) Sleep-related myoclonus in patients complaining of insomnia. Trans Am Neurol Assoc 100:19–22
Guilleminault C, Eldridge F, Dement W (1973) Insomnia with sleep apnea: a new syndrome. Science 181:856–858
Guilleminault C, Silvestri R, Coburn S, Dement WC, Cummiskey J (in press) Aging, breathing during sleep, and long-lasting benzodiazepines. Br J Clin Pharmacol
Harvey S (1980) Hypnotics and sedatives. In: Gilman A, Goodman L, Gilman A (eds) The pharmacological basis of therapeutics, 6th edn. MacMillan, New York
Hindmarch I, Clyde CA (1980) The effects of triazolam and nitrazepam on sleep quality, morning vigilance and psychomotor performance. Arzneim-Forsch 30:1163–1166
Hoddes E, Carskadon M, Phillips R, Zarcone V, Dement W (1972) Total sleep time in insomniacs. Sleep Research 1:152
Johnson L, Chernik D (1982) Sedative hypnotics and human performance. Psychopharmacology (Berlin) 76:101–113
Institute of Medicine (1979) Report of a study: Sleeping pills, insomnia, and medical practice. National Academy of Sciences, Washington DC
Kales A, Bixler EO, Soldatos CR, Vela-Bueno A, Caldwell AB, Cadieus RJ (1982) Biopsychobehavioral correlates of insomnia, part 1: role of sleep apnea and nocturnal myoclonus. Psychosomatics 23:589–600
Kales A, Scharf M, Kales J, Soldatos C (1979) Rebound insomnia: a potential hazard following withdrawal of certain benzodiazepines. JAMA 241:1692–1695
Kales A, Scharf M, Kales J (1978) Rebound insomnia: a new clinical syndrome. Science 201:1039–1041
Kales A, Caldwell A, Preston T, Healey S, Kales J (1976) Personality patterns in insomnia. Arch Gen Pschiat 33:1128–1134
Kleitman N (1963) Sleep and wakefulness. University of Chicago Press, Chicago
Krieger J, Mangin P, Kurtz D (1980) Les modifications respiratoires au cours du sommeil du sujet age normal. Rev EEG Neurophysiol 10:177–185
Kupfer D (1976) REM latency: a psychobiologic marker for primary depressive disease. Biol Pschiatr 11:159–174
Lavie P, Alroy G, Halpern E (1982) Apneic and nonapneic breathing disorders in sleep. Isr J Med Sci 18:523–533
Linnoila M, Erwin CW, Logue PE (1980) Efficacy and side effects of flurazepam and a combination of amobarbital and secobarbital in insomniac patients. J Clin Pharmacol 20:117–122
Lugaresi E, Coccagna G, Mantovani M, Berti-Ceroni G, Pazzaglia P, Tassinari C (1970) The evaluation of different types of myoclonus during sleep. Eur Neurol 4:321–331
Mattila J, Hammel R, Alexander B, Zustiak R (1977) Potential untoward effects of long-term use of flurazepam in geriatric patient. J Am Pharm Assoc 17:692–695
McGinty DJ, Arand DL, Littner MR (1981) Sleep-related breathing disorders in healthy and hypersomnolent older males. Sleep Research 10
Mendels J, Hawkins DR (1967) Sleep laboratory adaptation in normal subjects and depressed patients ("first night effect"). Electroencephalogr Clin Neurophysiol 22:556–558

Mendelson W, Garnett D, Gillin J (1981) Single case study: flurazepam induced sleep apnea syndrome in a patient with insomnia and mild sleep-related respiratory changes. J Nerv Ment Dis 169:261–264

Miles L, Dement W (1980) Sleep and aging. Sleep 3:119–220

Mitler M (1982) The multiple sleep latency test as an evaluation for excessive somnolence. In: Guilleminault C (ed) Sleeping and waking disorders: Indications and techniques. Addison Wesley, Palo Alto

Mitler M, Dement W (1981) Sleep disorders centers - for which patients? Consultant 21:155–164

Mitler MM, Seidel WF, Greenblatt DJ, van den Hoed J, Dement WC (in press) Simultaneous nighttime and daytime study of longterm treatment with triazolam, flurazepam and placebo. J Clin Pharmacother

Moldofsky H, Scarisbrick P, England R, Smythe H (1975) Musculoskeletal symptoms and non-REM sleep disturbance in patients with "Fibrositis syndrome" and healthy subjects. Psychosom Med 37:341–351

Monroe L (1967) Psychological and physiological differences between good and poor sleepers. J Abnorm Psychol 72:255–264

Nicholson AN, Stone BM, Pascoe PA (1982) Hypnotic efficacy in middleage. J Clin Psychopharmacol 2:118–121

Nicholson AN, Stone BM (1980) Activity of the hypnotics, flunitrazepam and triazolam, in man. Br J Clin Pharmacol 9:187–194

Oswald I, Adam K, Borrow S, Idzikowski C (1979) The effects of two hypnotics on sleep, subjective feelings and skilled performance. In: Passouant P, Oswald I (eds) Pharmacology of the states of alertness. Pergamon Press, New York

Rechtschaffen A, Kales A (eds), Berger R, Dement W, Jacobson A, Johnson L, Jouvet M, Monroe L, Oswald I, Roffwarg H, Roth B, Walter R (1968) A manual of standardized terminology, techniques, and scoring system for sleep stages of human subjects. U.S. Govt Printing Office, USPHS, Washington, DC

Richardson G, Carskadon M, Flagg W, van den Hoed J, Dement W, Mitler M (1978) Excessive daytime sleepiness in man: multiple sleep latency measurement in narcoleptic and control subjects. Electroencephagr Clin Neurophysiol 45:621–627

Roth T, Hartse KM, Saab PG, Piccione PM, Kramer M (1980) The effects of flurazepam, lorazepam, and triazolam on sleep and memory. Psychopharmacology (Berlin) 70:231–237

Roth T, Zorick F, Sicklesteel J, Stepanski E (1981) Effects of benzodiazepines on sleep and wakefulness. Br J Clin Pharm 11:31–35

Roth T, Zorick F, Wittig R, Roehrs T (1982) Pharmacological and medical considerations in hypnotic use. Sleep 5:46–52

Scharf MB, Kales A, Bixler EO (1975) Readaptation to the sleep laboratory in insomniac subjects. Psychophysiology 12:412–415

Schmidt HS, Kaelbling H (1971) The differential laboratory adaptation of sleep parameters. Biol Psychiatry 3:33–45

Seidel W, Dement WC (1982) Sleepiness in insomnia: evaluation and treatment. Sleep 5:182–190

Sherer M, Zarcone V, Kraemer H, Dement WC, van den Hoed J, Mitler MM (1981) Insomnia: Clinical and polysomnographic findings in patients presenting with the complaint of difficulty in initiating and maintaining sleep. Sleep Research 10:232

Smythe M, Giblin E, Lee K (1981) Prevalence of apneas and oxygen desaturation during sleep in healthy older men. Sleep Research 10:118

Spinweber CL, Johnson LC (1982) Effects of triazolam (0.5 mg) on sleep, performance, memory, and arousal threshold. Psychopharmacology 76:5–12

Symonds CP (1953) Nocturnal myoclonus. J Neurol Neurosurg Psychiatry 16:166–171

Webb W, Campbell S (1979) The first night effect revisited with age as a variable. Waking and Sleeping 3:319–324

Williams R, Hursch C, Karacan I (1972) Between-subject variability and night-to-night variability in insomniacs and normal controls. Sleep Res 1:154

Zorick F, Roth T, Hartse K, Piccione P, Stepanski E (1981) Evaluation and diagnosis of persistent insomnia. Am J Psychiatry 138:769–773

# Are Poor Sleepers Changed into Good Sleepers by Hypnotic Drugs?

K. Adam[1]

**Contents**



**Abstract**

Sleep can be measured by subjective ratings, electrophysiological recordings and by the physiological and biochemical changes occurring with sleep. Using these methods, we can select those who rate their sleep as unsatisfactory and those who feel fully satisfied by their sleep. Electrophysiological recordings of sleep show that there are relatively small differences between these good and poor sleepers: poor sleepers sleep less than good sleepers, but not as little as they think. However, the complaints of poor sleepers that they feel unrestored by their sleep should not be dismissed, for investigations employing the tools of physiology and biochemistry have revealed differences between good and poor sleepers that suggest that the sleep of poor sleepers may indeed be less restorative. The actions of hypnotic drugs on sleep can be similarly investigated. Preliminary findings suggest that hypnotic drugs may reverse some of the detrimental metabolic concomitants of poor sleep.

**Key Words**

Adrenaline/Benzoctamine/Blood pressure/Cortisol/Chlordiazepoxide/Chlormezanone/Diazepam/Flurazepam/Growth hormone/Heart rate/Lormetazepam/Nitrazepam/Noradrenaline/Oxygen consumption/Pentobarbitone/Sleep-wake cycle/Subjective and EEG measures.

---

1 Department of Psychiatry, University of Edinburgh, GB-Edinburgh, EH 10 5HF

Psychopharmacology Supplementum 1
Editors: I. Hindmarch, H. Ott and T. Roth

## 1 Introduction

Difficulty in falling asleep, waking too early, waking frequently, getting insufficient sleep, feeling tired and unrestored after a night's sleep – any or all of these complaints are voiced by those who call themselves poor sleepers. On the other hand, most hypnotic drugs hasten sleep, lengthen its duration and reduce the number of awakenings. But do hypnotic drugs change poor sleepers into good sleepers?

In this paper I shall be concerned with possible restorative processes of sleep, how these may be impaired in poor sleepers and how they may be affected by hypnotic drugs. First I shall describe the different methods by which sleep can be measured.

## 2 How Can Sleep Be Measured?

### 2.1 Subjective Ratings

The complaint of poor sleep is purely a subjective evaluation of the quality of sleep. We can attempt to find objective differences between good and poor sleepers, but the initial distinction is based upon their own opinions about their sleep. It is important to differentiate here between good and poor sleepers on the one hand and long and short sleepers on the other. The latter can be selected by objective criteria, the former only by their subjective reports. People have no difficulty in judging whether they are good or poor, heavy or light sleepers and can assess the quality of a night's sleep relative to usual. For example, according to the subjective ratings of volunteers, benzodiazepines such as lormetazepam and nitrazepam remain effective in improving sleep quality over many months of use (Oswald et al. 1982).

### 2.2 Electrophysiological Recordings

These recordings give us objective measures of sleep and enable us to make precise measurements of how long it takes a person to fall asleep, how many minutes they sleep, and how often and for how long they are awake during the night. In addition, EEG recordings have revealed that sleep is not a uniform state and it has been divided by international agreement into five stages (Rechtschaffen and Kales 1968). Sleep is broadly divided into two distinct phases: NREM or orthodox sleep, and REM or paradoxical sleep. These two phases of sleep alternate about five times through the night with a cycle length of around 100 min, and these sleep cycles display one of the ultradian rhythms exhibited in man of about this cycle duration.

REM sleep is characterized by jerky eye movements and loss of skeletal muscle tone punctuated by sporadic twitches. NREM or orthodox sleep is subdivided into four stages labelled 1, 2, 3 and 4. The number of minutes of stages 3 and 4 are usually combined and together are called slow-wave sleep (SWS), often thought of as the deepest kind of sleep. Slow-wave sleep and REM sleep have been thought particularly to be linked with the restorative processes of sleep (Oswald 1980). Confirmatory evidence for these beliefs has been provided by the third approach to the measurement of sleep.

### 2.3 Physiological Changes Associated with Sleep

It is possible to sample blood while a person sleeps: A venous catheter is inserted into the forearm vein and an extension tube attached, long enough to pass through the bedroom wall, allowing samples to be taken frequently without disturbing the sleeper. An important finding using this technique was the discovery that, in man, the large nocturnal output of growth hormone is dependent upon the presence of sleep and is particularly associated with slow-wave sleep (Sassin et al. 1969)

The minute by minute rates of oxygen consumption also can be measured and when correlated with the simultaneously recorded stages of sleep, human metabolic rate is found to be about 10% lower in stage 2 sleep than when recumbent but awake (Brebbia and Altshuler 1968; Haskell et al. 1981).

Heart rate, blood pressure and deep-body temperature all vary over the 24 hours and are at their lowest during the sleep period. Although the fall in core temperature, for example, is not sleep-dependent, it is lower during a night spent asleep than a night spent awake (Mills et al. 1978).

Just as sleep is associated with physiological changes so the converse is also true – changes in physiological processes can alter subsequent sleep.

### 2.4 Increased Metabolic Demand Changes Sleep

Hyperthyroid patients, with their raised metabolic rate, spend more of each night in SWS (Dunleavy et al. 1974). Even among euthyroid men, daytime levels of thyroxine correlate positively with the amount of SWS in the subsequent night (Johns et al. 1975).

Exercise greatly increases waking metabolic demand and following exercise men fall asleep more quickly (Browman 1980) and for longer (Moses et al. 1977). In athletes extra exercise by day leads to extra SWS by night (Shapiro et al. 1981), while my colleagues found that greater physical exercise in non-athletes led to greater nocturnal secretion of sleep dependent growth hormone and lowered overnight corticosteroids (Adamson et al. 1974).

Sleep deprivation increases metabolic demands and the first night of recovery sleep following sleep deprivation is not only of longer duration but also more time is spent in the deepest type of sleep – slow-wave sleep (Berger and Oswald 1962). All the above suggest that when extra metabolic demands are made there may be compensatory changes in sleep compatible with a belief that sleep has a role in recovery processes.

Not a single person has been found who does not sleep at all. Extravagant claims of not sleeping for years are made, but upon investigation are found to be untrue (Oswald and Adam 1980). So why do we spend so much of our lives asleep? The answers to this question provide some of the clues as to why some people are dissatisfied with their sleep, while others are content with their nightly quota.

## 3 Why Do We Sleep?

### 3.1 Biological Rhythms

The alternation between sleep and wakefulness is governed by an endogenous circadian rhythm: an in-built propensity to fall asleep at one time in the 24 h and awaken at another (Borbely 1982). All living creatures rest or sleep for part of each 24 h. The biological clock that drives the sleep-wake rhythm is most obvious when it is disturbed by trans-meridian jet travel or by shift work. Many of the problems of jet-travellers and shift-workers, sleep difficulties, mood changes and impaired performance, are a direct consequence of disturbing the sleep-wake rhythm (Mills 1973; Akerstedt and Torsvall 1978). It has been suggested that some poor sleepers have a sleep-wake cycle that is only weakly coupled to environmental time cues or that is permanently out of phase (Association of Sleep Disorders Centers 1979), thus leading to sleep difficulties akin to those experienced by jet-travellers or shift-workers. Certainly the artificial manipulation of the timing of sleep, to simulate time-zone changes, impairs people next day. For example, Taub and Berger (1974) have shown that shifting the sleep period for up to four hours earlier or later than normal leads to measurable deficits in performance and a poorer sense of well-being the next day.

Living things are not machines. They cannot be continuously active and working. But, unlike machines, living things repair their tissues and grow, and they mainly do this when they rest and sleep.

### 3.2 Sleep for Tissue Restoration and Growth

The recuperative value of sleep and its association with growth and repair has long been recognized (Oswald 1980). There are numerous animal studies that show that peak rates of cellular proliferative activity occur at the time of sleep (Adam 1980). In man the same association is found, e.g. our skin cells (Fisher 1968) and bone marrow cells (Mauer 1965) are replaced at a faster rate during the night. In growing boys, most ulnar bone growth occurs at night (Valk and van den Bosch 1978). Growth and repair necessarily depend upon net protein synthesis and therefore on a positive nitrogen balance. It has been found that more nitrogen is retained in humans deficient in growth hormone (GH) after an injection of GH at 2300 h, than after an identical injection given on another day at 0800 h, suggesting that the period of sleep following the 2300 h dose facilitated anabolic processes (Rudman et al. 1973). From these findings one would predict that lack of sleep or disturbed sleep would impair anabolism and so it is interesting that growth was retarded in children at times of disturbed sleep (Wolff and Money 1973).

The need for tissue renewal and growth is not confined to the growing phase of life. Adults too have to repair and replace their tissues which are undergoing perpetual, though not uniform, breakdown and renewal. Obvious examples are the skin and the gut lining. To put this in perspective, the entire lining of the gut is rubbed-off and replaced each 24 h (Leblond and Walker 1956). The replacement of these cells entails the synthesis of a considerable amount of new protein, and animal studies demonstrate that this replacement proceeds faster during the sleep phase (Adam 1980).

Not only is synthesis accelerated at the time of sleep but also, as described above, degradative metabolism is lowered by sleep for the rate of oxygen consumption is a direct measure of degradation. Whole body oxygen consumption rates in man are much lower at night than during a day of sedentary activities, and there is no overnight fall when subjects are denied sleep (Webb et al. 1980).

### 3.3 Detrimental Effects of Sleep Loss

These provide clues to the restorative role of sleep by the same line of reasoning used by endocrinologists when they investigate the function of a gland by observing the changes that follow its ablation.

Keeping 19 young men awake for two consecutive nights and days (on constant nitrogen intake throughout) led to a significant increase in nitrogen excretion on the second deprivation day (Scrimshaw et al. 1966). The negative nitrogen balance that ensued could be attributed to protein catabolic processes exceeding those of synthesis. After sleep deprivation, human muscle biopsies showed significant decreases in the activities of enzymes of energy metabolism and consequently lowered muscle efficiency (Vondra et al. 1981). Consistent with this finding is the impaired muscle power associated with sleep deprivation and its complete reversal following a night of recovery sleep (Copes and Rosenzweig 1972).

It is, though, mental functions that are particularly sensitive to sleep deprivation. The longer the time without sleep, the greater the pressure to sleep, suggesting some mounting deficit in cerebral repair and/or energy replenishment. Recovery can only be achieved by sleep, for bedrest is not a substitute for sleep in rejuvenating mental performance (Lubin et al. 1976). Animal studies have shown that sleep loss increases catabolic and decreases anabolic processes in the brain (Shapot 1957), leading to diminished concentrations of RNA and protein, effects that are reversed by subsequent sleep (Doemin and Rubinskaya 1974).

So staying awake when one should be asleep leads to impaired physical performance, poorer mood, and particularly impaired mental performance, coupled with a shift in the balance between synthesis and degradation, towards increased breakdown of protein. All the above suggest that the waking period is associated with a net loss of protein that is normally compensated for during sleep.

### 3.4 The Hormone Pattern Over the Sleep-Wake Cycle

By far the largest output of human growth hormone (GH) occurs during the early hours of sleep and is absolutely dependent upon the presence of sleep (Sassin et al. 1969). Merely lying in bed resting is insufficient to stimulate its release. In vivo, growth hormone has a number of well-established metabolic functions. It promotes general bodily growth and leads to positive nitrogen balance (Levine 1972) by stimulating the synthesis of RNA and protein and the uptake of amino acids into tissues (Korner 1965). In contrast, the circadian rhythms in the output of catabolic hormones, for example, adrenaline, noradrenaline and the corticosteroids, are entrained to the sleep-wake cycle such that peak levels occur during

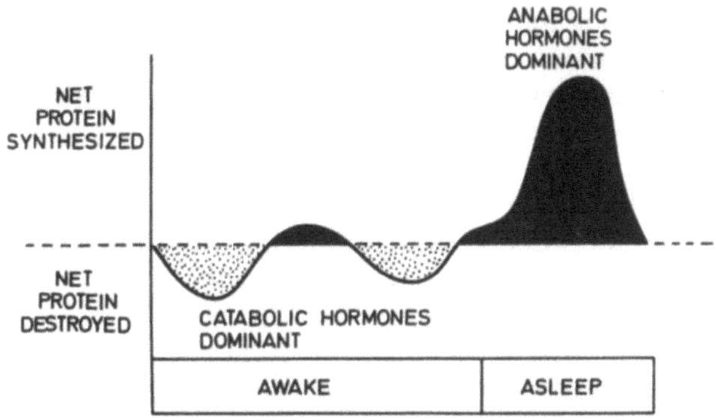


**Fig. 1.** Diagrammatic representation of the balance between the synthesis and degradation of protein in the body and the brain over the sleep-wake cycle

wakefulness and lowest outputs during the early hours of the customary sleep period (Weitzman et al. 1975). Though principally under circadian control the outputs of these catabolic hormones are reduced even further by being asleep (Weitzman et al. 1981). Corticosteroids reduce net protein synthesis (Tischler 1981) and so the low rates of output in the early hours of sleep come at the time when the levels of GH are maximal. Thus the hormone pattern of sleep, i.e. a combination of higher GH levels coupled with low levels of corticosteroids, promotes net protein synthesis during the sleep period, as the results of Rudman et al. (1973) indicated for humans.

In contrast, the high levels of adrenaline, noradrenaline and corticosteroids during the waking period promote catabolism and enable the organism to cope with the stresses and metabolic demands of waking activity.

I should stress though that it is not just the hormone pattern that accounts for sleep being associated with greater growth and faster repair. There are basic biochemical reasons why protein synthesis is accelerated during rest and sleep, and inhibited by the activities of wakefulness (Adam 1980). But the hormone pattern with sleep would help to ensure that sleep would be associated with sufficient net protein synthesis to make up for what had been lost during the waking period (Fig. 1).

But what about the people who complain of poor sleep – are they in fact less restored by their sleep?

## 4 What is Poor Sleep?

Poor sleep is a complaint of dissatisfaction with the quality of sleep. It is common, e.g. one study found that over 40% of respondents reported having a current or past problem with insomnia (Bixler et al. 1979), and the same conclusion could be drawn from the number of sleeping pills prescribed (Dunnell and Cartwright 1972). The prevalence of poor sleep depends upon the age and sex of those questioned, but broadly speaking the complaint of poor sleep increases with age and the incidence is higher in women. In a Scottish study about 40% of women over 45 years complained of being "light" sleepers and over 20% of women over

55 years thought that they usually took over one and a half hours to fall asleep (McGhie and Russell 1962). One American study reported that around 12% of adolescents questioned complained of chronic and severe sleep disturbances (Price et al. 1978) and another found that 20% of 18–30 year olds reported having difficulty in staying asleep, a figure that rose to well over 40% for those over 51 years of age (Bixler et al. 1979).

Objective recordings of sleep confirm that aging is associated with a reduction in total sleep and also with reduced amounts of slow-wave and REM sleep (Hayashi and Endo 1982). But there is wide variation among people of the same age and sex in the amount of time they sleep each night. Reported sleep durations among the population fall into an approximately normal distribution with the majority of people saying they sleep around 7 to 8 h (McGhie and Russell 1962; Palmer et al. 1980). Nevertheless, 15% of the respondents in the McGhie and Russell (1962) study said they slept for more than 9 h a night and 23% thought they slept for less than 6 h per night. Shorter than average sleep durations do not necessarily mean poor sleep. There are people who, though they only sleep two to three hours a night, are quite satisfied with their sleep (Jones and Oswald 1968). In any case it should not be assumed that subjective reports of lack of sleep will be borne out by objective measures of sleep.

### 4.1 Subjective and EEG Measures of Sleep in Good and Poor Sleepers

Among normal subjects it appears that there is reasonable agreement between their subjective estimates of how long it takes them to fall asleep and of how long they sleep when compared with objective recordings (Johns 1977; Frankel et al. 1978). However, those who describe themselves as poor sleepers significantly over-estimate how long they take to fall asleep and they under-estimate total sleep time (Frankel et al. 1978; Carskadon et al. 1976). Recently, with my colleague M. Tomeny, I have completed a study designed to compare those who describe themselves as poor or very poor sleepers with those who describe themselves as good or very good sleepers. We found that in the 18 middle-aged poor sleepers the average estimate of sleep latency over five consecutive nights was 51 min (range 13–137 min), whereas the EEG recordings showed that they took, on average, only 23 min to fall asleep (range 8–70 min). In contrast, the 18 matched good sleepers thought they took, on average, 23 min to fall asleep (range 8–43 min) which was not significantly different from the 16 minutes they actually took (range 8–41 min). There was in fact no significant difference between the goods and the poors in the EEG-recorded sleep latencies. The 18 poor sleepers had been individually matched with the 18 good sleepers for sex, age, height and weight and degree of over- and under-weight. This last factor, because I had previously found total sleep time to be correlated with the percentage by which a person's body weight deviates from the ideal for their height (Adam 1977 a). Though very closely matched for height and weight, the poor sleepers did sleep significantly less than the good sleepers (404 min v. 432 min). Both groups under-estimated total sleep time: the goods by 29 min and the poors by 63 min. Neither group thought their sleep, over the five laboratory nights, was significantly different from usual. The objectively recorded difference of 28 min between the goods and the poors is of the same order as in previous studies (Frankel et al. 1978; Monroe 1967) and appears insufficient to account for the dissatisfaction with sleep expressed by poor sleepers.

I earlier emphasized the importance of slow-wave sleep and REM sleep in recovery processes and so a possible explanation for poor sleepers' dissatisfaction could be that the "quality" of their sleep might be less in terms of the amount of SWS and REM sleep. So it is interesting that we found no differences between the goods and the poors for the number of mins of SWS (mean diff = 0.7 min) or REM sleep (mean diff = 1.3 min). These results are in contrast with previous reports of poor sleepers having less SWS (Frankel et al. 1978) or less REM sleep (Monroe 1967). However, in neither of these earlier studies had the subjects been matched for height and weight. I described above how quotas of SWS had been linked with metabolic differences and I have previously reported (Adam 1977b) and have recently confirmed that there is a positive correlation between the amounts of REM sleep and body weight.

The relatively small differences found between good and poor sleepers should not be taken to mean that poor sleepers are unjustified in their complaints, for the EEG cannot tell us if a minute of one person's sleep is worth as much as a minute of another person's sleep for recuperative processes. Indeed when awakened after five minutes of continuous sleep (by EEG criteria) poor sleepers are less likely to say they had been asleep than good sleepers (Borkovec et al. 1981). Perhaps the EEG misleads us in the case of these patients. We need other measures to understand better the complaints of poor sleepers.

## 4.2 Psychological and Biological Correlates of Poor Sleep

Monroe (1967) reported significant differences between good and poor sleepers on the MMPI (Minnesota Multi-Phase Personality Inventory) and Cornell Medical Index, and Tune (1969) found that introverts reported sleeping less than extroverts. Kales et al. (1976) similarly found that among insomniacs 85% had had one or more MMPI scales elevated above normal. The authors proposed that the internalization of psychological disturbance led to elevated emotional arousal and physiological activation and that this process underlies insomnia.

The complaint of poor sleep is also correlated with being of a nervous disposition (McGhie and Russell 1962), and we found that our poor sleepers scored significantly higher on scales measuring: neuroticism, anxiety, the somatic concomitants of anxiety and obsessionality and they were more pre-occupied with worries upon retiring to bed. Anxiety raises the metabolic rate (Landis 1925) and it increases the secretion of catabolic hormones such as adrenaline and cortisol. These are all factors that enhance degradative processes and tissue breakdown. Adrenaline also increases the rate of heat production (Boothby and Sandiford 1920) which may account for Monroe's (1967) poor sleepers having higher overnight rectal temperatures, while our own poor sleepers had significantly higher daytime oral temperatures. It must be supposed that these higher temperatures are sustained by higher rates of degradative metabolism in the poor sleepers.

Greater anxiety in poor sleepers may account for the findings of Johns et al. (1971) that poor sleepers had higher corticosteroids than good sleepers throughout the 24 hours. A similar, though non-significant difference between good and poor sleepers was present in our study.

In summary, poor sleepers sleep less than other people, but not as little as they think. They are more anxious, have higher body temperatures and may have higher outputs of the catabolic hormones adrenaline and cortisol. These differences in their metabolism suggest that poor sleepers have greater obstacles to recovery during sleep and may need more sleep than other people, but get less. Whether it is their anxious personalities that causes their chronic poor sleep or the other way round is not certain, but the associated heightened physiological arousal and increased catabolic hormone output suggest that their complaint of feeling unrestored by their sleep is in fact a true reflection of biochemical events.

## 5 Do Hypnotic Drugs Turn Poor Sleepers into Good Sleepers?

The EEG tells us that hypnotic drugs increase sleep duration and we know that many also reduce anxiety – so do they improve the restorative value of sleep in those who complain of poor sleep?

The EEG tells us nothing about the biochemical recovery processes occurring during sleep. Nor can it tell us if "drugged" sleep is as good as natural sleep. Many hypnotic drugs reduce the amounts of SWS (stages 3 and 4) and REM sleep recorded, the very stages of sleep that have been particularly linked with ideas about tissue restoration and repair – so one might wonder if the benefits of lengthened sleep when taking hypnotics could be offset by any detrimental effects of lost minutes of REM and SWS sleep. Yet poor sleepers certainly rate their sleep of higher quality when hypnotics are taken, such as chlormezanone, nitrazepam (Adam and Oswald 1982) and lormetazepam (Oswald et al. 1982). So one wonders if the greater satisfaction with their sleep when taking hypnotics would be reflected in measures of the restorative value of sleep? As yet this is a neglected area of sleep research but some inferences can be drawn. Raised corticosteroids (like raised adrenaline levels, higher temperatures and oxygen consumption rates) must reduce the restorative value of sleep, and it is interesting that many hypnotic drugs, which are equally useful as anxiolytics, are found to reduce corticosteroid output, for example chlordiazepoxide (Krulik and Cerny 1972), diazepam, nitrazepam and pentobarbitone (Oyama 1973) and benzoctamine (Ogunremi et al. 1973). However, many of the drugs reduce also the amounts of SWS sleep recorded. So the question arises, is the nocturnal secretion of growth hormone that is linked particularly with this type of sleep (Sassin et al. 1969) also diminished by hypnotic drugs? The available evidence suggests that this is not the case, because none among the following drugs reduced nocturnal growth hormone output: chlordiazepoxide, phenobarbitone (Takahashi et al. 1968; Prinz et al. 1981), nitrazepam (Adam et al. 1976), diazepam (Stokes et al. 1972; Tormey et al. 1979) or flurazepam (Rubin et al. 1973; Bixler et al. 1976). From these studies it appears that at least the benzodiazepine hypnotics do not interfere with the nocturnal growth hormone levels despite reducing SWS duration. It may be that these drugs merely interfere with the generation of the electrical brain waves without disturbing the biological processes associated with sleep.

Coupled with the knowledge that hypnotic drugs increase sleep duration, the studies above suggest that hypnotics such as benzodiazepines would be expected to push the balance between anabolic and catabolic processes towards greater anabolism. The only objective indication that this may be the case is the study of nitrogen balance before, during and after "therapeutic sleep" (Kuhn 1963), a technique in which patients are kept asleep for the majority of the 24 h by hypnotic drugs. During the period of induced sleep, patients were in positive nitrogen balance (so protein anabolic processes were outweighing those of protein breakdown), whereas before and after the drug treatment they were in negative nitrogen balance.

I believe that it will be the greater use of these more fundamental measures of sleep that will help us to understand better the complaint of poor sleepers that they feel unrestored by their sleep. One of the challenges of future research is to investigate the influence of hypnotic drugs on the biological processes that are normally facilitated by sleep and only then will we be able to answer the question "Are poor sleepers changed into good sleepers by hypnotic drugs?".

*Acknowledgements.* Thanks are due to the Scottish Hospital Endowments Research Trust and Schering AG (Berlin) for financial support of the study of good and poor sleepers.

## References

Adam K (1977a) Brain rhythm that correlates with obesity. Br Med J 2:234

Adam K (1977b) Body weight correlates with REM sleep. Br Med J 1:813–814

Adam K (1980) Sleep as a restorative process and a theory to explain why. Prog Brain Res 53:289–305

Adam K, Adamson L, Březinová V, Hunter WM, Oswald I (1976) Nitrazepam: lastingly effective but trouble on withdrawal. Br Med J 1:1558–1560

Adam K, Oswald I (1982) A comparison of the effects of chlormezanone and nitrazepam on sleep. Br J Clin Pharmacol 14:57–65

Adamson L, Hunter WM, Ogunremi OO, Oswald I, Percy-Robb IW (1974) Growth hormone increase during sleep after daytime exercise. J Endocrinol 62:473–478

Akerstedt T, Torsvall L (1978) Experimental changes in shift schedules – their effects on well-being. Ergonomics 21:849–856

Association of Sleep Disorders Centers (1979) Diagnostic classification of sleep and arousal disorders. Sleep 2:1–137

Berger RJ, Oswald I (1962) Effects of sleep deprivation on behaviour, subsequent sleep and dreaming. J Ment Sci 108:457–465

Bixler EO, Kales A, Santen R, Vela-Bueno A, Soldatos CR, Kotas KM (1976) Effects of flurazepam (Dalmane) on anterior pituitary secretion. Res Commun Chem Pathol Pharmacol 14:421–429

Bixler EO, Kales A, Soldatos CR, Kales JD, Healey S (1979) Prevalence of sleep disorders in the Los Angeles Metropolitan Area. Am J Psychiatry 136:1257–1262

Boothby WM, Sandiford I (1920) The effect of the subcutaneous injection of adrenaline chloride on the heat production, blood pressure and pulse rate in man. Am J Physiol 51:200–201

Borbely AA (1982) Sleep regulation: circadian rhythm and homeostasis. In: Ganten D, Pfaff D (eds) Sleep. Clinical and experimental aspects. Springer, Berlin Heidelberg New York 1:83–103

Borkovec TD, Lane TW, Van Oot PH (1981) Phenomenology of sleep among insomniacs and good sleepers: wakefulness experience when cortically asleep. J Abnorm Psychol 90:607–609

Brebbia DR, Altshuler KZ (1968) Stage related patterns and nightly trends of energy exchange during sleep. In: Kline NS, Laska E (eds) Computers and electronic devices in psychiatry. Grune and Stratton, New York, pp 319–335

Browman CP (1980) Sleep following sustained exercise. Psychophysiol 17:577–580

Carskadon MA, Dement WC, Mitler MM, Guilleminault C, Zarcone VP, Spiegel R (1976) Self-reports versus sleep laboratory findings in 122 drug-free subjects with complaints of chronic insomnia. Am J Psychiatry 133:1382–1388

Copes K, Rosenzweig J (1972) The effects of sleep deprivation upon motor performance of ninth-grade students. J Sports Med Phys Fitness 12:47–53

Doemin NN, Rubinskaya NL (1974) The protein and RNA content in neurons and their glial satellites of the rat brain supra-optic nucleus after REM sleep deprivation lasting 24 h. Doklady Academii Nauk SSSR 214:940–942

Dunleavy DLF, Oswald I, Brown P, Strong JA (1974) Hyperthyroidism, sleep and growth hormone. Electroenceph Clin Neurophysiol 36:259–263

Dunnell K, Cartwright A (1972) Medicine takers, prescribers and hoarders. Routledge and Kegan Paul, London

Fisher LB (1968) The diurnal mitotic rhythm in the human epidermis. Br J Dermatol 80:75–80

Frankel BL, Coursey RD, Buchbinder R, Snyder F (1978) Recorded and reported sleep in chronic primary insomnia. Arch Gen Psychiatry 33:615–623

Haskell EH, Palca JW, Walker JM, Berger RJ, Heller HC (1981) Metabolism and thermoregulation during stages of sleep in humans exposed to heat and cold. J Appl Physiol 51:948–954

Hayashi Y, Endo S (1982) All-night sleep polygraphic recordings of healthy aged persons: REM and slow-wave sleep. Sleep 5:277–283

Johns MW (1977) Validity of subjective reports of sleep latency in normal subjects. Ergonomics 20:683–690

Johns MW, Gay TJA, Masterton JP, Bruce DW (1971) Relationship between sleep habits, adrenocortical activity and personality. Psychosom Med 33:499–508

Johns MW, Masterton JP, Paddle-Ledinek JE, Patel YC, Winikoff D, Malinek M (1975) Variations in thyroid function and sleep in healthy young men. Clin Sci Mol Med 49:629–632

Jones HS, Oswald I (1968) Two cases of healthy insomnia. Electroenceph Clin Neurophysiol 24:378–380

Kales A, Caldwell AB, Preston TA, Healey S, Kales JD (1976) Personality patterns in insomnia. Arch Gen Psychiatry 33:1128–1134

Korner A (1965) Growth hormone control of biosynthesis of protein and ribonucleic acid. Recent Prog Horm Res 21:205–236

Krulík R, Černý M (1972) Influence of chlordiazepoxide on blood corticosterone under repeated stress. Acta Nerv Sup (Praha) 14:31–34

Kuhn E (1963) Protein metabolism during therapeutic sleep. Psychiat Neurol (Basel) 146:353–378

Landis C (1925) Metabolic rate during emotional reactions. Am J Physiol 74:188–203

Leblond CP, Walker BE (1956) Renewal of cell populations. Physiol Rev 36:255–276

Levine R (1972) Some mechanisms for hormonal effects on substrate transport. In: Hokin LE (ed) Metabolic pathways. Academic Press, London, 4:627–641

Lubin A, Hord DJ, Tracy ML, Johnson LC (1976) Effects of exercise, bed rest and napping on performance decrement during 40 hours. Psychophysiol 13:334–339

Mauer AM (1965) Diurnal variation of proliferative activity in human bone marrow. Blood 26:1–7

McGhie A, Russell SM (1962) The subjective assessment of normal sleep patterns. J Ment Sci 108:642–654

Mills JN (1973) Air travel and circadian rhythm. J R Coll Physicians, London, 7:122–131

Mills JN, Minors DC, Waterhouse JM (1978) The effect of sleep upon human circadian rhythms. Chronobiologica 5:14–27

Monroe LJ (1967) Psychological and physiological differences between good and poor sleepers. J Abnorm Psychol 72:255–264

Moses J, Lubin A, Naitoh P, Johnson LC (1977) Exercise and sleep loss: effects on recovery sleep. Psychophysiol 14:414–416

Ogunremi OO, Adamson L, Březinová V, Hunter WM, MacLean AW, Oswald I, Percy-Robb IW (1973) Two anti-anxiety drugs: a psychoneuroendocrine study. Br Med J 2:202–205

Oswald I (1980) Sleep as a restorative process: human clues. Prog Brain Res 53:279–288
Oswald I, Adam K (1980) The man who had not slept for 10 years. Br Med J 281:1684–1685
Oswald I, French C, Adam K, Gilham J (1982) Benzodiazepine hypnotics remain effective for 24 weeks. Br Med J 284:860–861
Oyama T (1973) Endocrine responses to anaesthetic agents. Br J Anaesth 45:276–281
Palmer CD, Harrison GA, Hiorns RW (1980) Sleep patterns and life style in Oxfordshire villages. J Biosoc Sci 12:437–467
Price VA, Coates TJ, Thoresen CE, Grinstead OA (1978) Prevalence and correlates of poor sleep among adolescents. Am J Dis Child 132:583–586
Prinz PN, Vitiello MV, Roehrs TA, Linnoila M, Weitzman ED (1981) Effect of phenobarbital on sleep and nighttime plasma growth hormone and cortisol levels. Can J Physiol Pharmacol 59:1139–1145
Rechtschaffen A, Kales A (1968) A manual of standardized terminology, techniques and scoring system for sleep stages of human subjects. National Institute of Health Publication, No. 204. Washington, D C: U.S. Government Printing Office
Rubin RT, Gouin PR, Arenander AT, Poland RE (1973) Human growth hormone release during sleep following prolonged flurazepam administration. Res Commun Chem Pathol Pharmacol 8:90–92
Rudman D, Freides D, Patterson JH, Gibbas DL (1973) Diurnal variation in the responsiveness of human subjects to human growth hormone. J Clin Invest 52:912–918
Sassin JF, Parker DC, Mace JW, Gotlin RW, Johnson LC, Rossman LG (1969) Human growth hormone release: relation to slow-wave sleep and sleep-waking cycles. Science 165:513–515
Scrimshaw NS, Habicht JP, Pellet P, Piche ML, Cholakos B (1966) Effects of sleep deprivation and reversal of diurnal activity on protein metabolism in young men. Am J Clin Nutr 19:313–319
Shapiro CM, Bortz R, Mitchell D (1981) Slow-wave sleep: a recovery period after exercise. Science 214:1253–1254
Shapot VS (1957) Brain metabolism in relation to the functional state of the central nervous system. In: Richter D (ed) Metabolism of the nervous system. Pergamon Press, London, pp 257–262
Stokes J, Chernik DA, Pandy G, Mendels J (1972) Effects of diazepam on growth hormone release during sleep. Sleep Res 1:190
Takahashi Y, Kipnis DM, Daughaday WH (1968) Growth hormone secretion during sleep. J Clin Invest 47:2079–2090
Taub JM, Berger RJ (1974) Acute shifts in the sleep-wakefulness cycle: effects on performance and mood. Psychosom Med 36:164–173
Tischler ME (1981) Hormonal regulation of protein degradation in skeletal and cardiac muscle. Life Sci 28:2569–2576
Tormey WP, Dolphin C, Darragh AS (1979) The effects of diazepam on sleep, and on the nocturnal release of growth hormone, prolactin, ACTH and cortisol. Br J Clin Pharmacol 8:90–92
Tune GS (1969) The influence of age and temperament on the adult human sleep-wakefulness pattern. Br J Psychol 60:431–441
Valk IM, Van den Bosch JSG (1978) Intra daily variation of the human ulnar length and short term growth – a longitudinal study in eleven boys. Growth 42:107–111
Vondra K, Broda V, Bass A, Kuhn E, Teisinger J, Anděl M, Veselková A (1981) Effects of sleep deprivation on the activity of selected metabolic enzymes in skeletal muscle. Eur J Appl Physiol 47:41–46
Webb P, Annis JF, Troutman SJ (1980) Energy balance in man measured by direct and indirect calorimetry. Am J Clin Nutr 33:1287–1298
Weitzman ED, Boyar RM, Kapen S, Hellman L (1975) The relationship of sleep and sleep stages to neuroendocrine secretion and biological rhythms in man. Recent Prog Horm Res 31:399–446
Weitzman ED, Zimmerman JC, Czeisler CA, Ronda J (1981) Cortisol secretion is inhibited during sleep in normal man. Sleep Res 10:107
Wolff G, Money J (1973) Relationship between sleep and growth in patients with reversible somatotrophin deficiency. Psychol Med 3:18–27

# Effects of Hypnotics in Insomniacs

# Psychological Performance Models as Indicators of the Effects of Hypnotic Drugs on Sleep

I. Hindmarch [1]

**Contents**



**Abstract**

A theoretical and practical scheme for the measurement of change in psychological performance is presented. An information processing paradigm is used as the basis for the model while personality, memory, motivational and experiential variables are shown to be amenable to control via the application of standard experimental methodologies.

The model is realised in practical experimental terms in the use of measures of choice reaction time and critical flicker fusion threshold. The reliability and sensitivity of these parsimonious indices of performance change is illustrated in a brief review of the effects of benzodiazepine hypnotics on early morning performance.

**Key Words**

Benzodiazepines/Behavioural hangover/Choice reaction time/Critical flicker fusion threshold/Flunitrazepam/Flurazepam/Leeds Sleep Evaluation Questionnaire/Loprazolam/Lorazepam/Lormetazepam/Midazolam/Nitrazepam/Temazepam/Trait and state performance/Triazolam.

## 1 Introduction

The study of any aspect of human experience and behaviour achieves psychological relevance only when viewed within the context and framework of a well-designed model or conceptual system. Little attention has been given by most researchers to the theoretical basis of the performance measures they use to assess

1 Human Psychopharmacology Research Unit, University of Leeds, GB-Leeds, LS2 9JT

Psychopharmacology Supplementum 1
Editors: I. Hindmarch, H. Ott and T. Roth

the activity of hypnotic drugs on sleep and related behaviours. The lack of a structural notion of the nature of the behaviour to be measured has led to a profusion of idiosyncratic definitions of performance and a plethora of psychological tests purporting to measure it.

Consistency in the use of the expression "psychological performance" is difficult to find in the literature as different authors have totally different conceptions as to the meaning of the term. Skill, competence, attention, vigilance, stimulus detection, manual dexterity, sensorimotor co-ordination, mental ability, abstract reasoning, problem solving, concept formation, remembering and forgetting, learning, motor control and even, at an epistemological level, understanding have all, at some time or another, been used as synonymous with "psychological performance"

It is, of course, essential to decide when drawing up a model of performance whether the intention is to make an absolute measure of performance reflecting some essential behavioural trait, or, whether the need is for a performance measure sensitive to a change of state on some aspect of behaviour. It does not always follow that the model used as a theoretical basis for "trait performance" will be appropriate when sensitivity to a change of "state performance" is required.

As this paper is primarily concerned with the change in aspects of sleep and early morning performance brought about by the administration of hypnotic drugs, we will develop only those models of performance relating to the detection of change of state.

## 2 Experimental Methodology

### 2.1 Choice of the Performance Task

The major assumption of the psychopharmacologist is that the effects of a psychoactive drug will manifest as a change in the performance of an appropriate overt behavioural activity. However, the performance task must be carefully chosen and decided on with due consideration of the theoretical model otherwise any observed drug effects might be too task or situation specific to be of any general use in estimating the effects of a particular drug on behaviour.

Changes in proof-reading ability (Adams 1974); the absolute auditory threshold (Van Houten and Zenhausern 1967); short and long term memory (Ghoneim and Mewaldt 1977); the discrimination conditioning of the eyelid response (Gupta 1974); the speed of recognition of hidden words (Stitt et al. 1977); the duration of visual afterimages (Malpas and Joyce 1969); saccadic eye movements (Aschoff et al. 1975); a rudder control test (Gagné and Fleishman 1959) and the speed of putting caps onto ballpoint pens (Lahtinen et al. 1978) have been produced by a range of psychotropic compounds.

However, without the benefit of a theoretical framework against which to view these various effects such isolated, specific and discrete findings can tell us little about the general nature of the change in psychological performance brought about by the administration of psychoactive drugs.

The relationship between overt performance and the physical and psychological stimulation impinging upon an individual at any moment in time is necessarily complex but a parsimonious model must be developed if measures of psychological performance are to achieve pragmatic or heuristic usefulness in studying sleep and related behaviour.

## 2.2 Information Processing of Performance

The simplest model of performance identifies stimulus (S) and response (R) as the only important variables to be considered. Although SR models of performance are widely used by experimental psychologists working with animals, they are too simplistic to account for the diversity of the human organism's response to environmental stimulation. The inclusion of the organism (O) as a mediating influence between S and R, to produce the well-known SOR model of behaviour (Osgood 1953), is an important advance on the simple model for it allows some account to be taken of the effects of personality, motivation, memory, prior learning and experience on the co-ordination of stimulus and response systems. The mediating function of the organism is rarely constant with respect to time because of the great intra-individual variation in the temporal activity of cognitive and affectual systems. Furthermore, as Brunswik (1943) has indicated, our sensory impressions have, at best, only an adequate correlation with the original stimulus and our responses are only a reflection of the way an individual has utilised a proportion of the cues available. Hammond (1966) and Hammond and Joyce (1975) have developed the mathematical basis of Brunswik's arguments to provide measures of decision-making ability, judgmental processing skills and cognitive performance which, although outside the scope of this paper, provide an exemplary instance of the development of tests of performance based on reasoned theoretical arguments.

An adaption of Brunswik's Lens model, to show how psychomotor performance is dependent upon the adequate processing and utilisation of stimulus and response information, is presented in Fig. 1.

This diagram also illustrates the vicarious nature of the mediation provided by the organism's cognitive, i.e. brain and central nervous system, functioning and shows that for optimal levels of performance it is necessary to achieve correlation coefficients ($r$) for both cue utilisation and cue processing relationships as close to unity as possible.

Psychological performance is a reflection of the competence with which the stimulus and response cues are utilised and co-ordinated. In complex performance tasks, e.g. driving a motor vehicle, the sensory and motor cues are not instantly recognisable and much learning and experience of the validity of the various cues must take place before sensorimotor co-ordination and, ultimately, behavioural competence can be achieved. It follows then, that any test measure of performance must employ simple stimulus-recognition and motor-response components if the effects of learning and experience are to be avoided or, at least, minimised. The use of parsimonious test measures does not obviate, as we shall see later, the necessity for an adequate experimental methodological control of learning effects, via the training of all subjects on all test measures.

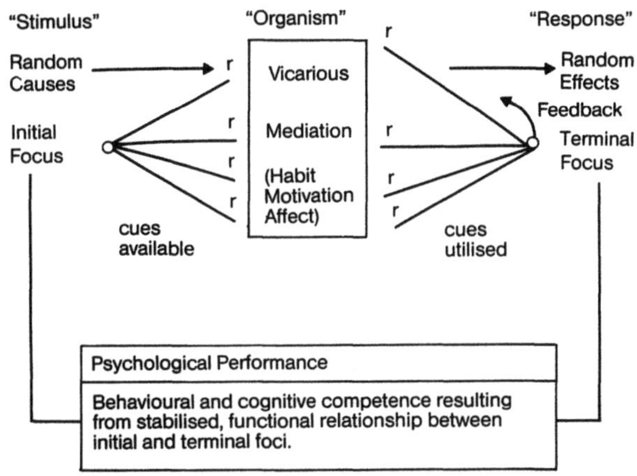


**Fig. 1.** A free adaptation of Brunswik's Lens model illustrates the probabilistic nature of the relationship between initial and terminal foci. Psychological performance is regarded as the behavioural and cognitive competence which results from a stabilised, functional co-ordination of stimulus and response

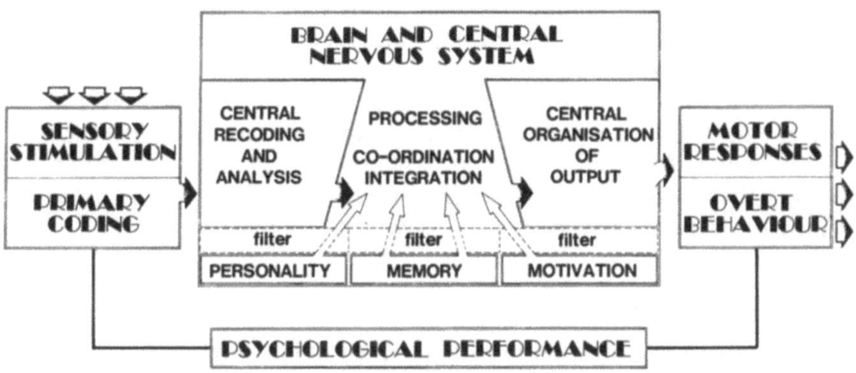


**Fig. 2.** Personality, motivation and memory play their part in influencing the co-ordination of the information flow between sensory stimulation and motor responses via the brain and central nervous system. Performance is regarded as the achievement of a close integrated concordance between stimulus and response systems

Having realised an information processing model of performance, the task is now to present this model in experimental, i.e. test measure or assessment, techniques. It has to be emphasised that if the psychopharmacological effects of hypnotics are to be measured with any degree of psychological relevance, then the study of the effects of such drugs within the context of a well-defined model of behaviour must be consistently pursued (Michon 1976).

The information flow, intrinsic to the Brunswik model, between stimulus and overt behavioural response is illustrated in Fig. 2.

In this figure the co-ordination of stimulus and response necessary for the optimal level of performance is seen to be dependent upon the activity of the brain and central nervous system. It is also obvious that the level of arousal and activation of the brain will be partly determined by the influence of personality, motivation and memory.

## 3 Psychopharmacological Studies

### 3.1 Personality Variables

Eysenck (1963, 1972) and Claridge (1967, 1970) have shown that an inverted U relationship holds between some personality dimensions, e.g. neuroticism, and performance on sensorimotor tasks like the pursuit rotor. The inverted U relationship implies that high neuroticism subjects will have poorer performance than less neurotic ones, because of their personality. Inter-individual differences in performance, due to personality, are well-illustrated in the different psychomotor test scores which have been observed in patient and "normal" volunteer populations (Malpas et al. 1974; Tansella et al. 1974). Janke et al. (1979) and Debus (1981) have further demonstrated the theoretical and practical importance of observing differences in performance due to inter-subject differences in personality and CNS arousal. In psychopharmacological studies it is not always necessary to measure the extent to which such variables affect performance. It is, however, always necessary to control and exclude such sources of variability by the application of proper experimental methodologies. In practice this is relatively easy to effect as personality variables have a more pronounced effect at the extremes of affectual dimensions. All studies, both in patients and volunteers, should minimise the influence of inter-subject variation in trait personality by pre-selecting and screening on standard psychometric assessments.

### 3.2 Motivational Factors and Learning Effects

Motivational factors can affect the results obtained in performance studies. The intentions of volunteers, the level of payment of subjects and the expectation of the experimenter and subject can all have a profound influence on experimental results (Ayd 1972). These extraneous variables can only be controlled by the use of double-blind experimental designs, a careful screening of volunteers, the use of experienced experimenters and a thoroughly reasoned protocol to govern the pragmatics of the test situation.

The intrinsic motivation of the task situation is an important determinant of performance. Drug action on a performance measure can also be affected by the nature of the assessment task, but the sensitivity of the performance measure can be ensured by including a verum, or positive internal control, in the drug treatment regimen. For example, amylobarbitone sodium is known to have sedative effects. If such effects are not obvious on an assessment measure following the experimental use of the drug, then it must be assumed that the test is insensitive and no credence can be given to any findings obtained in such an instance.

Any test of psychomotor performance involving the co-ordination of sensory and motor systems, e.g. the pursuit rotor, will be prone to practice and learning effects as, on repeated administration, the subject acquires the skills that facilitate performance. Practice, learning and the effects of memory on performance measures are relatively easy to control. Prior to entry in a study relying on a sensorimotor measure of performance all subjects must be trained on the task until their "learning curve" has reached a plateau, i.e. until the response measure has reached a limiting value and maintained such a value for several trials. When subjects are trained to a criterion, where no further increase in performance can be detected, they can then be admitted to a study. Such pre-training can completely eliminate learning effects, as evidenced in the unchanging placebo condition responses found in a model study by Täuber et al. (1979).

Personality, memory and motivation are still going to influence performance although they can be viewed as relatively unimportant, when the intention is to measure a change in performance, as the variables can be isolated "outside the model" by the proper application of standard experimental procedures.

### 3.3 Psychomotor Performance

We can now proceed to examine the realisation of the model in terms of tests of psychological performance (Fig. 3) shown to be sensitive to the effects of psychoactive drugs (Hindmarch 1980).

Such a realisation enables the identification of the different aspects of psychomotor performance and the contribution of sensory, central and motor processes. A battery of tests, including those assessing each of the three components of performance, is the usual way to assess a change in psychomotor ability. The effects of psychoactive drugs are likely to be observed in a change in CNS function and it has been argued (Holmberg 1981; Hindmarch 1981) that the Critical

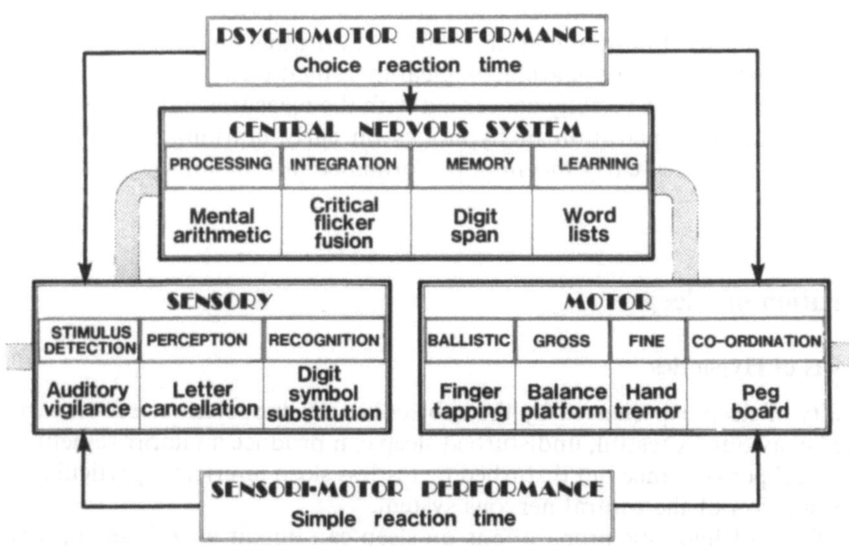


**Fig. 3.** Tests of performance which have been shown to be a sensitive index of the activity of psychotropic drugs (adapted from Hindmarch, 1980)

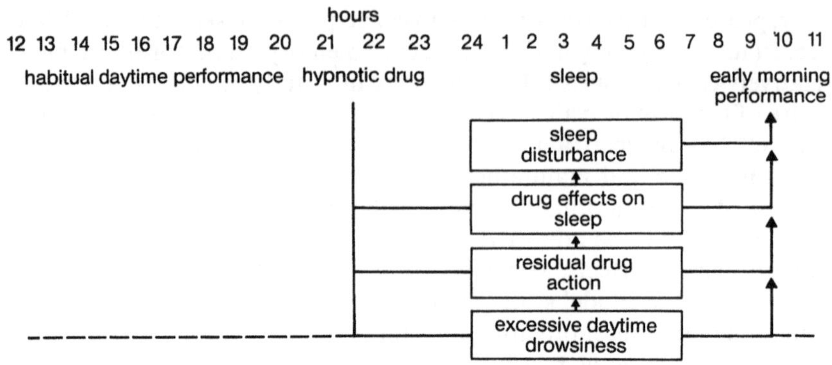


**Fig. 4.** The various factors affecting early morning performance following the nocturnal administration of hypnotics

Flicker Fusion Threshold represents the most reliable, objective measure. An indirect index of CNS activity of psychotropic drugs can be obtained from a choice reaction time task providing that the motor component of the task is measured separately from the total reaction time. Such a modus operandi enables the measurement of the stimulus processing and central integrative aspects of the task by the simple expedient of subtracting the motor time from the total response latency. As long as the stimulus recognition task is not difficult then it can readily be assumed that total reaction time minus motor movement time is equivalent to CNS processing latency. An apparatus (the Leeds Psychomotor Tester from ZAK GmbH, Simbach/Inn, FRG) for the measurement of motor and CNS processing times in a choice reaction time situation has been developed (Hindmarch 1975, 1980, 1981; Hindmarch and Parrott 1978a, 1978b; Hindmarch and Clyde 1980a, 1980b; Hindmarch et al. 1980) as a portable apparatus for use in volunteer and patient psychopharmacological investigations.

In this paper we are especially concerned with the measurement of the effects of the nocturnal administration of hypnotics on early morning performance. Hypnotics can influence early morning performance in 4 major ways as Fig. 4 illustrates.

## 4 Evaluation of Sleep

### 4.1 Effects of Hypnotics

The quality of sleep experienced by the subject has an important effect on early morning behaviour. A restful, undisturbed sleep can produce an improvement of psychological performance but disturbed or restless sleep interferes, particularly, with the function of the central nervous system.

The effects of hypnotic preparations on sleep can impair as well as improve early morning performance. Many effective sleep inducers will necessarily produce a "hangover" of behavioural disruption the next morning. Tables 1 and 2

**Table 1.** Leeds sleep evaluation questionnaire values (mm) after acute nocturnal administration of a benzodiazepine, compared to placebo baselines

| | | Leeds sleep evaluation questionnaire factors | | | |
|---|---|---|---|---|---|
| | | Getting to sleep (GTS) | Quality of sleep (QOS) | Awakening from sleep (AFS) | Behaviour following wakefulness (BFW) |
| Nitrazepam | 2.5 mg | + 2.5 | + 1.6 | − 0.9 | 0.0 |
| | 5.0 mg | + 6.6 | + 12.1 [a] | − 12.6 [b] | − 5.8 [a] |
| | 10.0 mg | + 18.0 [a] | + 22.0 | − 8.0 [b] | − 5.0 [b] |
| Flurazepam | 15.0 mg | + 6.5 [a] | + 10.4 [a] | − 7.9 [a] | − 0.1 |
| Flunitrazepam | 1.0 mg | + 16.0 [c] | + 0.2 | − 3.0 | − 5.5 |
| Lormetazepam | 2.0 mg | + 4.0 [a] | − 1.0 | − 4.0 | − 3.0 |
| Loprazolam | 0.5 mg | + 9.3 [a] | + 15.5 [c] | − 3.4 | − 25.9 [c] |
| Temazepam | 20.0 mg | + 17.4 [c] | + 17.0 [b] | + 3.2 | − 0.2 |

[a] $p < 0.05$; [b] $p < 0.01$; [c] $p < 0.001$

**Table 2.** Leeds sleep evaluation questionnaire values (mm) after repeated nocturnal administration of a benzodiazepine, compared to placebo baselines

| | | Leeds sleep evaluation questionnaire factors | | | |
|---|---|---|---|---|---|
| | | Getting to sleep (GTS) | Quality of sleep (QOS) | Awakening from sleep (AFS) | Behaviour following wakefulness (BFW) |
| Nitrazepam | 5.0 mg | − 0.4 | + 10.3 | − 11.9 [b] | − 6.9 [b] |
| | 10.0 mg | + 14.0 [b] | + 16.0 | − 16.0 [c] | − 7.0 [c] |
| Flurazepam | 15.0 mg | + 13.0 [d] | + 16.7 [c] | − 5.0 [b] | − 1.3 |
| Flunitrazepam | 1.0 mg | + 26.0 [d] | − 2.4 | − 6.2 | − 5.1 |
| Lorazepam | 3.0 mg | + 29 [b] | + 13.0 | − 14.0 [b] | − 22.0 [b] |
| Lormetazepam | 2.0 mg | + 14.0 [c] | + 10.0 [c] | − 3.0 | − 5.0 |
| Loprazolam | 1.0 mg | + 14.5 [c] | + 13.5 [c] | − 13.9 [d] | − 16.6 [d] |
| Temazepam [a] | 20.0 mg | + 24.6 [c] | + 20.0 [c] | + 7.4 | + 5.0 |
| | 40.0 mg | + 30.7 [c] | + 25.0 [c] | − 2.9 | + 1.0 |
| | 60.0 mg | + 31.7 [c] | + 24.0 [c] | + 0.9 | + 1.7 |
| Triazolam | 0.5 mg | + 22.0 [c] | + 18.0 [b] | − 14.0 [b] | + 1.0 |

[a] Measures taken in patients; [b] $p < 0.05$; [c] $p < 0.01$; [d] $p < 0.001$

present data from studies using the Leeds Sleep Evaluation Questionnaire to evaluate the subjective response to drug treatment.

Hypnotic preparations which reduce REM sleep can often be shown to produce a rebound of impaired performance following cessation of treatment. The relationship between the changes in the architecture of sleep stages brought about by hypnotic drugs and subsequent changes in performance is not yet fully understood, and it is often difficult to distinguish between the changes brought about

**Table 3.** Effects of acute nocturnal doses of benzodiazepines on next morning measures of psychomotor performance (with respect to placebo controls)

| | | Choice reaction time [ms] | Critical flicker fusion threshold [Hz] |
|---|---|---|---|
| Nitrazepam | 2.5 mg | − 16 | − 0.4 |
| | 5.0 mg | + 30 | − 0.5 |
| | 10.0 mg | + 42 ($p < 0.02$) | − 1.3 |
| Flunitrazepam | 1.0 mg | + 11 | − 0.1 |
| Lormetazepam | 0.5 mg | − 13 | + 0.1 |
| | 1.0 mg | + 12 | − 0.5 |
| | 2.0 mg | − 5 | − 0.6 |
| Loprazolam | 0.5 mg | − 20 ($p < 0.001$) | − 0.3 |
| | 1.0 mg | + 10 | − 0.5 |
| | 2.0 mg | 0 | 0 |
| Temazepam | 10.0 mg | + 2 | + 0.2 |
| | 20.0 mg | + 4 | + 0.2 |
| | 30.0 mg | + 22 ($p < 0.05$) | − 1.1 ($p < 0.05$) |
| | 40.0 mg | + 27 ($p < 0.0001$) | No data |
| | 60.0 mg | + 9 ($p < 0.05$) | No data |
| Triazolam | 0.5 mg | − 27 | + 1.0 |
| Midazolam | 5.0 mg | − 18 | 0 |
| | 10.0 mg | − 20 | 0 |
| | 15.0 mg | + 7 | 0 |
| | 20.0 mg | + 34 | 0 |

**Table 4.** Effects of repeated nocturnal doses of benzodiazepines on next morning measures of psychomotor performance (with respect to placebo controls)

| | | Choice reaction time [ms] | Critical flicker fusion threshold [Hz] |
|---|---|---|---|
| Nitrazepam | 5.0 mg | + 11 ($p < 0.05$) | − 0.1 |
| | 10.0 mg | + 15 ($p < 0.02$) | − 0.6 |
| Flunitrazepam | 1.0 mg | + 33 | No data |
| Flurazepam | 15.0 mg | No data | − 1.0 |
| Lormetazepam | 0.5 mg | − 14 | + 0.3 |
| | 1.0 mg | − 12 | 0 |
| | 2.0 mg | + 3 | + 0.5 |
| Loprazolam | 0.5 mg | − 10 | + 0.5 |
| | 1.0 mg | 0 | − 0.2 |
| Temazepam | 10.0 mg | + 5 | − 0.1 |
| | 20.0 mg | + 8 | − 0.2 |
| | 30.0 mg | + 20 ($p < 0.05$) | − 1.0 ($p < 0.05$) |
| | 40.0 mg | + 22 ($p < 0.001$) | + 0.2[a] |
| | 60.0 mg | + 3 | + 0.1[a] |
| Triazolam | 0.5 mg | − 14 | + 1.0 |

[a] Data from patient population

by direct residual pharmacological activity from those indirect changes in performance resulting from drug-induced changes in sleep variables.

### 4.2 Residual Pharmacological Activity

Residual pharmacological activity due directly to the presence of the drug or its active metabolites can disrupt early morning performance. Furthermore, residual daytime drowsiness, leading to naps and short daytime sleeps, can produce sleep induction problems at night. It is easy to see how a vicious circle can develop where the sleep problem is a direct result of the residual activity of the hypnotic used to promote sleep.

The problem of identifying the source of the residual activity of hypnotic drugs is, again, one of experimental methodology and the proper use of placebo and verum controlled designs. A discussion of trial methodology is outside the scope of this paper but the usefulness of the model detailed here and realised in choice reaction time and critical flicker fusion measures is illustrated in the two tables (Tables 3 and 4) summarising the early morning activity of a range of benzodiazepine hypnotics given the night before. All the studies reviewed are placebo controlled and utilise similar methodologies and treatment regimens. In this context these tables are not offered other than to show the usefulness of the realisation of this particular model of performance via Choice Reaction Time and Critical Flicker Fusion Threshold in discrimination of the effects of different drugs on early morning psychological performance.

## References

Adams RG (1974) Pre-sleep ingestion of two hypnotic drugs and subsequent performance. Psychopharmacologia (Berlin) 40:185–190

Aschoff JC, Becker W, Weinert D (1975) Computer analysis of eye movements: evaluation of the state of alertness and vigilance after supiride medication. J Pharmac Clin 11:93–97

Ayd FJ (1972) Motivations and rewards for volunteering to be an experimental subject. Clin Pharmacol Ther 13:771–781

Brunswik E (1943) Organismic achievement and environmental probability. Psychol Rev 50:255–272

Claridge GS (1967) Personality and Arousal. Pergamon, Oxford

Claridge GS (1970) Drugs and Human Behaviour. Allen Lane, London

Debus G (1981) Models of the connection between sedation, relaxation and performance. Clobazam. Academic Press, London, pp 43–49

Eysenck HJ (1963) Experiments with drugs. Pergamon, Oxford

Eysenck HJ (1972) Handbook of abnormal psychology. Pitman Medical, London

Gagné RM, Fleishman EA (1959) Psychology and human performance. Holt, New York

Ghoneim MM, Mewaldt SP (1977) Studies on human memory: the interaction of diazepam, scopolamine and physostigmine. Psychopharmacology 52:1–6

Gupta BS (1974) Stimulant and depressant drugs on kinaesthetic figural after-effects. Psychopharmacologia (Berlin) 36:275–280

Hammond KR (1966) The psychology of Egon Brunswik. Holt, Rinehart, Winston, London

Hammond KR, Joyce CRB (1975) Psychoactive drugs and social judgement: Theory and Research. John Wiley and Sons, London

Hindmarch I (1975) A 1,4-benzodiazepine, temazepam (K 3917): its effect on some psychological parameters of sleep and behaviour. Arzneim Forsch/Drug Res 25(II):1836–1839

Hindmarch I (1980) Psychomotor function and psychoactive drugs. Br J Clin Pharmacol 10:189–209
Hindmarch I (1981) Measuring the effect of psychoactive drugs on higher brain function. Advances in human psychopharmacology. JAI Press, Connecticut 2:99–127
Hindmarch I, Clyde CA (1980a) The effects of triazolam and nitrazepam on sleep quality, morning vigilance and psychomotor performance. Arzneim Forsch/Drug Res 30(II):1163–1166
Hindmarch I, Clyde CA (1980b) A preliminary investigation of the effects of a 1,4-benzodiazepine derivative (HR158) on subjective aspects of sleep and objective measures of early morning performance. Drugs Exptl Clin Res 2(2):61–70
Hindmarch I, Parrott AC (1978a) A repeated dose comparison of the side effects of five antihistamines on objective assessments of psychomotor performance, central nervous system, arousal and subjective appraisal of sleep and early morning behaviour. Arzneim Forsch/Drug Res 28(1):483–486
Hindmarch I, Parrott AC (1978b) The effect of a sub-chronic administration of three dose levels of a 1,5-benzodiazepine clobazam on subjective aspects of sleep and psychomotor performance the morning after nighttime medication. Arzneim Forsch/Drug Res 28(II):2169–2172
Hindmarch I, Parrott AC, Stonier PD (1980) The effects of nomifensine and HOE 8476 on car driving and related psychomotor performance. Roy Soc Med Int Cong Symp Series 25:48–54
Holmberg G (1981) Critical Flicker Fusion (CFF) test for sedative effects of antidepressants. Acta Psychiatr Scand [Suppl] 290, 63:289–301
Janke W, Debus G, Longo N (1979) Differential psychopharmacology of tranquillising and sedating drugs. Differential psychopharmacology of anxiolytics and sedatives, vol 14. Karger, Basel, pp 13–98
Lahtinen U, Lahtinen A, Pekkola P (1978) The effect of nitrazepam on manual skill, grip strength and reaction time with special reference to subjective evaluation of effects of sleep. Acta Pharmacol Tox 42:130–134
Malpas A, Joyce CRB (1969) Effects of nitrazepam, amylobarbiton and placebo on some perceptual, motor and cognitive tasks in normal subjects. Psychopharmacologia (Berlin) 14:167–177
Malpas A, Legg NJ, Scott DF (1974) Effects of hypnotics on anxious patients. Br J Psychiatry 124:482–484
Michon JA (1976) Human information processing – with and without drugs. Psychiat Neurol Neurochir (Ams) 76:163–174
Osgood CE (1953) Method and theory in experimental psychology. Oxford University Press, New York
Stitt FW, Latour R, Frane JW (1977) A clinical study of naproxen-diazepam drug interaction on tests of mood and attention. Curr Ther Res 21:149–156
Täuber K, Badian M, Brettel HF, Royen T, Rupp W, Sittig W, Uihlein M (1979) Kinetic and dynamic interaction of clobazam and alcohol. Br J Clin Pharmacol 7:91–97
Tansella M, Zimmerman-Tansella C, Lader M (1974) The residual effects of N-desmethyldiazepam in patients. Psychopharmacologia 138:81–90
Van Houten PL, Zenhausern R (1967) Meprobamate and absolute auditory threshold. J Aud Res 7:253–257

# Sleep Laboratory Study of Lormetazepam in Older Insomniacs

G. W. Vogel[1]

**Contents**



## Abstract

Lormetazepam is a new benzodiazepine hypnotic. Previous work has indicated that lormetazepam has an intermediate to short elimination half-life, i.e. in the range of 5–15 h. Hence, in older patients, the drug should be safe and hypnotically active in doses equal to or less than the doses recommended for young adults. The present study tested this hypothesis. We studied ten healthy subjects, aged 55 and older, with both subjective and objective insomnia. Subjective insomnia was the complaint of requiring at least 45 min to fall asleep and sleeping less than six and a half hours per night.

Each complaint was present on at least 50 % of the nights for at least three months. Objective insomnia was measured polysomnographically and was present on at least two of the last three nights of four consecutive nights of placebo baseline. The study involved a design in which treatment was administered in a double-blind fashion. Each subject was studied for 14 consecutive nights in the sleep laboratory. The drug was administered for seven consecutive nights which were preceded by a placebo baseline and followed by a placebo period of drug withdrawal. On each laboratory night subjects were monitored by continuous, all-night conventional EEG/EOG/EMG recordings. Each laboratory morning subjects completed a questionnaire on which they rated six characteristics of their sleep on the previous night. At study entry and again at study end, each subject had a physical examination by a Board internist and clinical laboratory tests. Each laboratory morning and evening subjects had a screening physical exam and completed an 11-item hypnotic drug side-effect questionnaire and a 56-item review of medical systems questionnaire. Compared with the median baseline night, on the median drug night lormetazepam 0.5 mg significantly increased total sleep time by about 25 min. The drug's reductions of sleep latency were substantial. In addition, lormetazepam 0.5 mg significantly decreased number of awakenings. No objective evidence was found of either tolerance developing to the hypnotic efficacy of lormetazepam 0.5 mg or of rebound insomnia.

1 Georgia Mental Health Institute and Department of Psychiatry, Emory University School of Medicine, Atlanta, GA 30306, USA

Psychopharmacology Supplementum 1
Editors: I. Hindmarch, H. Ott and T. Roth

**Key words**

Awakenings/Benzodiazepine hypnotic/Carryover effect/Convulsive disorders/Delta sleep/Depth of sleep/EEG/Elimination half-life/EMG/EOG/Hypersensitivity to benzodiazepines/Hypnotic efficacy/Nocturnal myoclonus/NREM sleep/Psychiatric disorder/Rebound insomnia/Refreshing quality of sleep/REM sleep/Sleep apnea/Sleep latency/Tolerance.

## 1 Introduction

Lormetazepam is a new benzodiazepine hypnotic. Previous work has indicated that lormetazepam has an intermediate to short elimination half-life, i.e. in the range of 5–15 h (Greenblatt et al. 1982). This finding suggests that its metabolic biotransformation will be "relatively uninfluenced by old age" (Greenblatt et al. 1981). Hence, in older patients, the drug should be safe and hypnotically active in doses equal to or less than the doses recommended for young adults. The present study tested this hypothesis. A dose of 1.5 or 2 mg has been found to have significant hypnotic effects in healthy adults younger than 55 or 60 years (Heidrich et al. 1981; Vogel, unpublished study). We present data here on the safety and hypnotic efficacy of lormetazepam 0.5 mg in healthy insomniacs aged 55 and older.

## 2 Methods

We studied ten healthy subjects, aged 55 and older, with both subjective and objective insomnia. Subjective insomnia was the complaint of requiring at least 45 min to fall asleep and the complaint of sleeping less than six and a half hours per night. Each complaint was present on at least 50% of the nights for at least three months. Objective insomnia was measured polysomnographically and was present on at least two of the last three nights of four consecutive nights of placebo baseline. We defined objective insomnia to be median (of baseline nights 2–4) wake time of at least 45 min during a 480-min nocturnal polygraphic recording.

The ten subjects included 2 males and 8 females with a mean age of 60 years (range = 55 to 71 years). Subjects were healthy, as assessed by prestudy medical history and physical examination (performed by a Board internist), and as assessed by prestudy clinical laboratory tests (CBC, SMA-12, urinalysis, and 12-lead ECG). We excluded subjects (1) with a history of drug abuse, alcohol abuse, or addiction; (2) with a history of serious psychiatric disorder; (3) with hepatic, renal, metabolic, or convulsive disorders; (4) with hypersensitivity to benzodiazepines; and (5) with established diagnosis of sleep apnea or nocturnal myoclonus. We excluded subjects who (6) were grossly under- or over-weight; or (7) were taking psychoactive medication (e.g., sedatives, antidepressants, tranquilizers), antihistamines, narcotics, or any drug which would interfere with the evaluation of the safety or efficacy of lormetazepam. We excluded subjects who (8) had received any benzodiazepines or other hypnotic or psychoactive drugs within ten days (30 days for barbiturates) prior to study entry. Finally, we excluded (9) women of childbearing potential not practicing a medically acceptable method of birth control, pregnant females, and nursing mothers.

The study involved a design in which treatment was administered in a double-blind fashion. Each subject was studied for 14 consecutive nights in the sleep laboratory. The schedule was as follows: night 1, placebo (adaptation); nights 2–4, placebo (baseline); nights 5–11, drug (lormetazepam 0.5 mg); nights 12–14, placebo (withdrawal). Thus, the drug was administered for seven consecutive nights which were preceded by a placebo baseline and followed by a placebo period of drug withdrawal.

On each laboratory night, treatment (lormetazepam 0.5 mg tablet or identically appearing placebo tablet) was administered orally exactly 30 min before "lights out" bedtime. Each subject's bedtime (clock time of retirement) was the same on all the subject's 14 laboratory nights and an attempt was made to set each subject's laboratory bedtime near the subject's usual home bedtime. On each laboratory night total polygraphic recording time was 480 min.

On each laboratory night subjects were monitored by continuous, all night conventional EEG/EOG/EMG (polygraphic) recordings. The recordings, identified only by random code numbers, were scored by technicians according to standard Rechtschaffen-Kales criteria (1968).

The following polygraphic efficacy variables were scored: total sleep time; % sleep (% of total time in bed occupied by sleep); wake time in each third of the night; stage 1 sleep latency (time from "lights out" to the onset of first half-minute of stage 1 sleep); stage 2 sleep latency (time from "lights out" to the onset of first half-minute of stage 2 sleep); persistent sleep latency (time from "lights out" to the onset of the first sleep that persisted for at least ten consecutive minutes); mid-wake time (wake time between persistent sleep onset and last half-minute of any sleep stage); and number of awakenings > 15 s duration.

The following polysomnographic sleep stage variables were scored: sleep stages 1, 2, delta, and REM (in minutes and in percent of total sleep time); REM latency (duration of all NREM sleep preceding first half-minute of stage REM sleep); movement time, and total polygraphic recording time (total lab time).

We also measured efficacy subjectively. Each laboratory morning subjects completed a questionnaire on which they rated six characteristics of their sleep in the previous night. The questions concerned time to fall asleep, number of awakenings, duration of sleep, time of final awakening, depth of sleep, and refreshing quality of sleep.

Safety was assessed in several ways. At study entry and again at study end each subject had a physical examination by a Board internist and had the following clinical laboratory tests: CBC, SMA-12, urinalysis, and a 12-lead ECG. Each laboratory morning and evening subjects had a screening physical exam. This consisted of supine and standing blood pressure, supine and standing pulse, oral temperature, and neurologic tests for coordination and balance (finger-nose coordination, straight-line walk, and Romberg). Finally, each laboratory morning and evening subjects completed an 11-item hypnotic drug side-effect questionnaire and a 56-item review-of-medical-systems questionnaire.

In our statistical analysis matched pair t-tests were used to assess differences in polygraphic variables and in vital signs. Wilcoxon matched pair, signed rank tests were used to assess differences in subjective sleep-efficacy variables and in subjective adverse effects. Baseline-drug period differences in efficacy variables (polygraphic and subjective) were assessed by one-tailed tests. All other differences were assessed by two-tailed tests. For all variables we used Siegel's median as the measure of central tendency (Siegel 1956).

## 3 Results

### 3.1 Polygraphic Efficacy Variables

The main polygraphic efficacy results are summarized in Table 1.

Compared with the median baseline night, on the median drug night lormetazepam 0.5 mg significantly increased total sleep time by about 25 min (and significantly decreased total wake time by the same amount; $p < 0.01$). However, the drug did not significantly change baseline total sleep time on the first or last (7th) drug night ($p > 0.10$). The hypnotic effects of lormetazepam 0.5 mg were strongest in the first third of the night. Compared with the median baseline night, on the first, median, and last drug nights lormetazepam 0.5 mg significantly decreased wake time in the first third of the night ($p < 0.05$). Wake time in the middle third of the night was not decreased by lormetazepam 0.5 mg, probably because its baseline value was very small. In the last third of the night lormetazepam 0.5 mg tended to decrease wake time ($p < 0.10$) on the median drug night, but not on the first or last drug nights.

Compared with the median baseline night, on the first, median, and last drug nights lormetazepam 0.5 mg significantly decreased all three measures of sleep latency ($p < 0.05$). The drug's reductions of sleep latency were substantial, viz, from median baseline levels of about 30 to 45 min to drug-period levels of about 17 to 24 min, respectively.

The drug had no significant effect on one measure of sleep maintenance, viz, wake time between persistent sleep onset and last steep of the night. But it did improve another measure of sleep maintenance, viz, number of awakenings. Compared with median baseline night, on the first, median and last drug nights, lormetazepam 0.5 mg significantly decreased number of awakenings.

We assessed the possible development of tolerance to the hypnotic effects of the drug by comparing first and last (7th) drug night values of each efficacy variable. We found no significant difference between first and last drug night values in any polygraphic efficacy variable. Thus, we found no objective evidence that over seven consecutive nights of lormetazepam 0.5 mg administration, tolerance developed to the hypnotic efficacy of lormetazepam 0.5 mg.

We assessed possible drug-withdrawal rebound insomnia and possible drug-withdrawal hypnotic "carryover effects" by comparing baseline median values of efficacy variables with their values on post-drug night 1 and on the median post-drug night. We found no significant difference between baseline and first post-drug night values of efficacy variables. Thus, we found no evidence that withdrawal from a week of nightly administration of lormetazepam 0.5 mg produced a rebound insomnia or a hypnotic carryover.

**Table 1.** Polygraphic efficacy

| | BSL MDN | Drug NT 1 | Drug NT 7 | Drug MDN | P-Drug NT 1 | P-Drug MDN |
|---|---|---|---|---|---|---|
| *Total sleep time* | 389.0 | 403.1 | 410.0 | 413.4 | 357.0 | 379.1 |
| P (difference from BSL) | | NS | NS | c | NS | NS |
| P (difference from Drug NT 1) | | | NS | | | |
| *Total wake time* | 89.2 | 73.0 | 67.2 | 64.5 | 120.0 | 98.2 |
| P (difference from BSL) | | NS | NS | c | NS | NS |
| P (difference from Drug NT 1) | | | NS | | | |
| *Wake time by thirds of night* | | | | | | |
| First third | 49.2 | 34.6 | 26.4 | 28.2 | 61.7 | 47.2 |
| P (difference from BSL) | | b | c | c | NS | NS |
| P (difference from Drug NT 1) | | | NS | | | |
| Second third | 11.8 | 10.0 | 17.4 | 12.3 | 24.2 | 15.6 |
| P (difference from BSL) | | NS | NS | NS | NS | NS |
| P (difference from Drug NT 1) | | | NS | | | |
| Final third | 25.9 | 28.3 | 23.4 | 16.7 | 34.2 | 27.4 |
| P (difference from BSL) | | NS | NS | a | NS | NS |
| P (difference from Drug NT 1) | | | NS | | | |
| *Wake time between PSTNT sleep onset and last sleep* | 40.0 | 48.3 | 43.6 | 33.8 | 52.8 | 47.5 |
| P (difference from BSL) | | NS | NS | NS | NS | NS |
| P (difference from Drug NT 1) | | | NS | | | |
| *Stage 1 latency* | 31.5 | 16.8 | 18.8 | 18.6 | 33.8 | 27.6 |
| P (difference from BSL) | | c | b | c | NS | NS |
| P (difference from Drug NT 1) | | | NS | | | |
| *Stage 2 latency* | 35.4 | 21.0 | 21.8 | 22.3 | 37.8 | 34.5 |
| P (difference from BSL) | | c | b | c | NS | NS |
| P (difference from Drug NT 1) | | | NS | | | |
| *PSTNT sleep latency* | 45.1 | 24.6 | 21.4 | 23.8 | 51.4 | 38.2 |
| P (difference from BSL) | | b | b | b | NS | NS |
| P (difference from Drug NT 1) | | | NS | | | |
| *Number of awakenings* | 18.8 | 14.2 | 13.7 | 15.2 | 16.8 | 15.5 |
| P (difference from BSL) | | b | b | c | NS | a |
| P (difference from Drug NT 1) | | | NS | | | |

*Key:* Probability of difference between baseline and each post-baseline variable (e.g. Drug NT 1) is indicated in the row under each post-baseline variable. Probability of difference between Drug night 1 and Drug night 7 is indicated under Drug night 7. MDN is median
NS: Not significant at 0.10
[a] Probability < 0.10; [b] Probability < 0.05; [c] Probability < 0.01

Using the baseline, drug, and post-drug means instead of medians, we repeated all the above statistics on the polygraphic efficacy variables. The results were essentially the same except in two instances. Compared with baseline means (but not compared with baseline medians), on the first and last (7th) drug nights, lormetazepam 0.5 mg significantly increased total sleep time and significantly decreased total wake time.

### 3.2 Polygraphic Sleep Stages

Stage 1 sleep was not affected by lormetazepam 0.5 mg on the first drug night, median drug night, or last drug night. However, on the first post-drug night stage 1 sleep (in minutes and percent of total sleep time) was greater than on the median baseline night. On the median post-drug night stage 1 sleep was not significantly different than on the median baseline night.

Stage 2 sleep (in minutes but not in percent of total sleep time) was significantly increased over its baseline value by lormetazepam 0.5 mg throughout the week of drug administration. Specifically, compared with median baseline values, stage 2 minutes were increased on the first, median, and last drug nights ($p < 0.05$). Baseline and post-drug values of stage 2 sleep were not significantly different.

Delta sleep was significantly decreased during lormetazepam nights. Specifically, compared with baseline median values, delta sleep (in minutes and percent) was significantly decreased on the first drug night and median drug night but not on the last drug night. Baseline and post-drug values of delta sleep were not significantly different.

REM sleep (in minutes and percent of sleep time) was not affected by lormetazepam 0.5 mg. Specifically, compared with baseline median values, REM sleep was not significantly different on the first drug night, median drug night, last drug night, first post-drug night, or median post-drug night. REM latency was also not affected by lormetazepam 0.5 mg.

Finally, movement time was not affected by lormetazepam 0.5 mg.

Using baseline, drug night and post-drug night means instead of medians, we repeated all the above statistics on sleep stage variables. With minor differences the results were essentially the same by both techniques.

### 3.3 Subjective Efficacy Variables (Table 2)

Compared with the median baseline night, on the median drug night, subjectively (i.e. by questionnaire response) lormetazepam 0.5 mg decreased time to fall asleep, increased duration of sleep, decreased number of awakenings, and increased depth of sleep. All these subjective effects were significant at $p < 0.05$ except the increase of depth of sleep which was significant at $p < 0.10$. Except for the decrease of sleep latency, these effects were observed on the first drug night. None of the subjective effects were observed on the last drug night. Lormetazepam 0.5 mg had no effect on the final awakening and it improved the refreshing quality of sleep only on the first drug night.

We assessed possible subjective post-drug rebound insomnia and possible subjective post-drug carryover hypnotic effects by comparing baseline and post-drug values of the six subjective efficacy variables. We found no significant difference between median baseline night and first or median post-drug nights in the subjective efficacy variables. Thus, we found no evidence that withdrawal from seven consecutive nights of lormetazepam 0.5 mg produced a subjective rebound insomnia or a subjective carryover effect.

We assessed possible subjective tolerance to the efficacy of lormetazepam 0.5 mg by comparing each subjective efficacy variable on drug night one and on drug night seven. We found no significant first-seventh drug night differences in

**Table 2.** Subjective efficacy

| | BSL MDN | Drug NT 1 | Drug NT 7 | Drug MDN | P-Drug NT 1 | P-Drug MDN |
|---|---|---|---|---|---|---|
| *Time to fall asleep* | 3.7 | 3.4 | 3.3 | 3.3 | 4.0 | 3.7 |
| *P* (difference from BSL) | | NS | NS | [b] | NS | NS |
| *P* (difference from Drug NT 1) | | | NS | | | |
| Meaning of entries | 1 Less than 15 min | | | | | |
| | 2 15–30 min | | | | | |
| | 3 30–45 min | | | | | |
| | 4 45–60 min | | | | | |
| | 5 More than 60 min | | | | | |
| *Number of awakenings* | 3.1 | 1.7 | 2.0 | 1.9 | 2.1 | 2.2 |
| *P* (difference from BSL) | | [b] | NS | [b] | NS | NS |
| *P* (difference from Drug NT 1) | | | NS | | | |
| *Duration of sleep* | 3.1 | 3.6 | 3.4 | 3.4 | 2.8 | 3.0 |
| *P* (difference from BSL) | | [b] | NS | [b] | NS | NS |
| *P* (difference from Drug NT 1) | | | NS | | | |
| Meaning of entries | 1 Less than 4 h | | | | | |
| | 2 4–5 h | | | | | |
| | 3 5–6 h | | | | | |
| | 4 6–7 h | | | | | |
| | 5 More than 7 h | | | | | |
| *Final awakening* | 2.1 | 2.2 | 2.5 | 2.1 | 2.5 | 2.4 |
| *P* (difference from BSL) | | NS | NS | NS | NS | NS |
| *P* (difference from Drug NT 1) | | | NS | | | |
| Meaning of entries | 1 At end of lab time | | | | | |
| | 2 1–15 min before end | | | | | |
| | 3 15–30 min | | | | | |
| | 4 30–60 min | | | | | |
| | 5 1–2 h | | | | | |
| | 6 More than 2 h | | | | | |
| *Depth of sleep* | 4.2 | 4.5 | 4.2 | 4.6 | 3.6 | 3.6 |
| *P* (difference from BSL) | | [a] | NS | [a] | NS | NS |
| *P* (difference from Drug NT 1) | | | NS | | | |
| Meaning of entries | 1 Extremely light | | | | | |
| | 2 Very light | | | | | |
| | 3 Light | | | | | |
| | 4 Average | | | | | |
| | 5 Deep | | | | | |
| | 6 Very deep | | | | | |
| | 7 Extremely deep | | | | | |
| *Refreshing quality of sleep* | 4.2 | 4.5 | 3.8 | 4.3 | 3.3 | 4.0 |
| *P* (difference from BSL) | | [b] | NS | NS | NS | NS |
| *P* (difference from Drug NT 1) | | | NS | | | |
| Meaning of entries | 1 Extremely bad | | | | | |
| | 2 Very bad | | | | | |
| | 3 Bad | | | | | |
| | 4 Average | | | | | |
| | 5 Good | | | | | |
| | 6 Very good | | | | | |
| | 7 Extremely good | | | | | |

*Key:* Probability of difference between baseline and each post-baseline variable (e.g. Drug NT 1) is indicated in the row under each post-baseline variable. Probability of difference between Drug night 1 and Drug night 7 is indicated under Drug night 7. MDN is median
NS: Not significant at 0.10
[a] Probability $< 0.10$; [b] Probability $< 0.05$; [c] Probability $< 0.01$

subjective efficacy variables. Thus, we found no evidence that subjective tolerance to the hypnotic efficacy of lormetazepam 0.5 mg developed over seven consecutive nights of administration.

All of the above statistical tests, which were done using medians of subjective efficacy variables, were repeated using means. The results were exactly the same.

## 4 Safety

There were no clinically important differences in the prestudy and end study physical exams by the Board internist or in prestudy and end study clinical laboratory tests (CBC, SMA-12, urinalysis, and 12-lead ECG).

Lormetazepam 0.5 mg had no clinically important effects on the daily screening neurological examinations and on the daily vital signs. Nevertheless, at various times during the week of drug administration lormetazepam 0.5 mg did produce slight, but statistically significant, effects on some vital signs. Evening oral temperature was slightly decreased ($p < 0.05$). Evening standing systolic blood pressure and morning standing and supine systolic and diastolic blood pressure were reduced by small but significant amounts. Morning pulse was slightly, but significantly, increased. All other vital signs were not significantly different from baseline during the week of drug administration ($p > 0.05$). There were also small, but statistically significant, effects on vital signs at various times during the period of drug withdrawal. Morning oral temperature was slightly decreased. There was a small decrease in evening blood pressure (both supine and standing) and in morning supine blood pressure. All other vital signs were not significantly different during the baseline and post-drug periods. None of the significant differences in vital signs produced clinical symptoms.

The eleven items on the morning and evening subjective (hypnotic) adverse effect questionnaire were not significantly different on the median baseline night and on drug nights or on post-drug nights. Also the 56-item review-of-medical-systems questionnaire, which was completed each morning and each evening, showed no clinically significant adverse effects of lormetazepam 0.5 mg. Occasionally or infrequently, mild symptoms were noted on this form. These included the following: on the mornings following drug administration five subjects occasionally noted mild headache, four subjects occasionally noted mild nasal congestion, three subjects occasionally noted mild drowsiness, and two subjects infrequently noted dry mouth. Other symptoms were noted less frequently and almost always were mild (i.e., rated 1 on a 0–3 point scale of severity).

## 5 Discussion

We found that, measured both subjectively and objectively (polygraphically), lormetazepam 0.5 mg was an efficacious hypnotic in subjects aged 55 years and older.

On the median treatment night the drug significantly reduced both the subjective experience of sleep latency and the three objective (polygraphic) measures of sleep latency. The effects on objective sleep latency were large and persisted from the first to the seventh (last) drug night. The reduction of subjective sleep latency, though present on the median drug night, was not significant on the first or last drug night.

Lormetazepam 0.5 mg also increased both subjective and objective sleep time. The subjective increase of sleep time began on the first drug night. There was a discrepancy about when the objective (polygraphic) increase of sleep time began. In comparison with the mean baseline night, but not in comparison with the median baseline night, total sleep time increased on the first drug night. The discrepancy arose because mean baseline total sleep time was less than median baseline total sleep time.

The hypnotic effects of lormetazepam 0.5 mg appear to be strongest in the early part of the night. In particular, its effects in reducing wake time were significant in the first third of the night, not significant in the middle third, and only intermittently significant in the last third of the night. Also, the drug had no significant effect on wake time between persistent sleep onset and last sleep of the night. Both objectively and subjectively, the drug decreased number of awakenings throughout its week of administration.

We found no evidence, either polygraphically or subjectively, of a rebound insomnia. This finding contrasts with other reported data. Oswald et al. (1979) found a rebound insomnia following withdrawal of lormetazepam. Also lormetazepam is reported to have an intermediate duration elimination half-life (Greenblatt et al. 1982). Hence, the absence of rebound insomnia in our studies contrasts with evidence in other studies that rebound insomnia is often produced by benzodiazepine hypnotics with short or intermediate elimination half-lives (Kales et al. 1979).

We found no polygraphic or subjective evidence of a carryover hypnotic effects during withdrawal from the drug.

We found no polygraphic or subjective evidence of tolerance to the drug's hypnotic effects over seven consecutive nights of its administration. This result has also been found in other studies (Heidrich et al. 1981; Vogel, unpublished study; Oswald et al. 1979).

Like other benzodiazepines (Vogel et al. 1976; Kay et al. 1976), the drug increased stage 2 sleep and decreased delta sleep. The drug had no effect on REM sleep. In clinically high doses other benzodiazepines decrease REM sleep (Kay et al. 1976). Hence, the absence of any effect on REM sleep by lormetazepam 0.5 mg may be a function of the low dose or may be a relatively unusual characteristic of the drug. During its week of adminstration the drug had no effect on stage 1 sleep, but there was a significant increase of stage 1 sleep on the first post-drug night. This may be the only indication in our study of some tendency toward a rebound insomnia on drug withdrawal.

Other than mild and occasional possible adverse effects (such as morning drowsiness, headache, nasal congestion, and dry mouth), we found no adverse effects of lormetazepam 0.5 mg. Thus, we found the drug to be safe as assessed by pre and post study physical examinations and clinical laboratory tests (CBC, urinalysis, SMA-12, and 12-lead ECG); twice daily administered 11-item hypnotic drug side-effects questionnaire and 56-item review-of-medical-systems questionnaire; and by twice daily screening physicals for vital signs, balance, and coordination.

In summary, we found that lormetazepam 0.5 mg was a safe and efficacious hypnotic when administered for seven consecutive nights to healthy, older insomniacs. Its strongest hypnotic effects appear to be in the first part of the night. In our study the drug did not produce rebound insomnia or clinically significant adverse effects.

## References

Greenblatt DJ, Divoll M, Abernathy DR, Shader RI (1982) Benzodiazepine hypnotics: kinetic and therapeutic options. Sleep 5:S18–S27

Greenblatt DJ, Shader RI, Divoll M, Harmatz JS (1981) Benzodiazepines: a summary of pharmacokinetic properties. Br J Clin Pharmacol 11:115–165

Heidrich H, Ott H, Beach RC (1981) Lormetazepam – a benzodiazepine derivative without hangover effect? A double-blind study with chronic insomniacs in a general practice setting. Int J Clin Pharmacol Ther Tox 19:11–19

Kales A, Scharf M, Kales J, Soldatos C (1979) Rebound insomnia: A potential hazard following withdrawal of certain benzodiazepines. JAMA 241:1692–1695

Kay DC, Blackburn AB, Buckingham JA, Karacan I (1976) Human pharmacology of sleep. In: Williams RL, Karacan I (eds) Pharmacology of sleep. John Wiley and Sons, New York, pp 83–210

Oswald I, Adam K, Borrow S, Idzikowski C (1979) The effect of two hypnotics on sleep, subjective feelings, and skilled performance. In: Passouant P, Oswald I (eds) Pharmacology of the states of alertness. Pergamon Press, Oxford, New York, pp 51–63

Rechtschaffen A, Kales A (eds) (1968) A manual of standardized terminology, techniques and scoring system for sleep stages of human subjects. Public Health Service, U.S. Government Printing Office, Washington, DC

Siegel S (1956) Nonparametric statistics for the behavioral sciences. McGraw-Hill Book Company, New York, p 25

Vogel GW Unpublished study

Vogel GW, Barker K, Gibbons P, Thurmond A (1976) A comparison of the effects of flurazepam 30 mg and triazolam 0.5 mg on the sleep of insomniacs. Psychopharmacologia 47:81–86

# Effects of Two Benzodiazepines on the Speed and Accuracy of Perceptual-Motor Performance in the Elderly

K. Morgan[1]

**Contents**



**Abstract**

The daytime performance efficiency of 12 elderly subjects of average age 81.5 years (range 75–96 years) was examined in a cross-over study following lormetazepam 1 mg, nitrazepam 5 mg, and placebo capsules nightly for 7 nights. Performance was assessed on the Gibson spiral maze, and a reciprocal tapping task. In both tasks the speed and the accuracy of performance were independently measured. Performance testing sessions were conducted on the morning following the first, and the morning following the seventh dose of each of the three experimental treatments.

Performance on the Gibson spiral maze showed no significant effect of either of the active drugs. On the reciprocal tapping task, speed was similarly unaffected by both drugs. However, while neither drug significantly affected overall accuracy after the first dose, nitrazepam but not lormetazepam significantly impaired overall accuracy after seven consecutive doses. This difference between nitrazepam and lormetazepam was significant. Further analyses showed nitrazepam consistently to be associated with impaired accuracy at both intermediate and high levels of task complexity. Lormetazepam, on the other hand, was associated with impairment only at the highest level of task complexity. The overall pattern of impairment associated with nitrazepam, but not with lormetazepam, was consistent with drug accumulation.

**Key Words**

Accumulation/Clifton assessment procedures/Gibson spiral maze/Lormetazepam/Nitrazepam/Reciprocal tapping task/Task complexity.

## 1 Introduction

Research findings indicate that, relative to younger age groups, elderly individuals are more sensitive to the residual effects of long-acting, cumulative hypnotic drugs (Castleden et al. 1977; Swift et al. 1981). The present investigation was

1 Department of Psychiatry, University of Edinburgh, GB-Edinburgh, EH10 5HF

Psychopharmacology Supplementum 1
Editors: I. Hindmarch, H. Ott and T. Roth

therefore undertaken to evaluate and compare the effects of nitrazepam 5 mg and lormetazepam 1 mg on the daytime performance of elderly volunteers. Performance was assessed on tasks known to be sensitive to residual effects of both high (Salem et al. 1982) and low (Morgan 1982) dose nitrazepam in the elderly. The study design required a period of drug taking which would allow cumulative effects, if present, to emerge.

## 2 Subjects

Subjects (nine females and three males) were resident within Local Authority Homes for the Elderly in the Edinburgh area. None was receiving psychoactive medication, and each abstained from alcohol for the duration of the study. All subjects were in good general physical health, and the mental competence of each was assessed on the Clifton Assessment Procedures for the Elderly (Pattie and Gilleard 1975) prior to their inclusion in the study.

## 3 Design and Method

Identical matching capsules of placebo, lormetazepam 1 mg, and nitrazepam 5 mg were supplied by Schering Chemicals Limited. Subjects received each of these treatments for a period of seven nights, in a balanced double-blind sequence. Each of the seven treatment nights were preceded by two nights of placebo capsules. Thus, subjects received capsules continuously for 27 nights. A practice session followed the second placebo capsule at the start of the experiment, and thereafter subjects were tested on the morning following the first, and the morning following the seventh capsule within each drug week. The performance tests, which took approximately 20 min to complete, included:

*The Gibson Spiral Maze* (Gibson 1978); this paper and pencil test requires the subject to track through a simple spiral maze as quickly, and as accurately, as possible. Three measures were recorded:

i) the time taken to complete the maze;
ii) the number of errors made while completing the maze; and
iii) the total efficiency score, calculated as time × log (error + 1)

*A Reciprocal Tapping Task* (Morgan 1982); in which the subject is required to tap two identical circular targets placed 10 inches apart (centre to centre) alternately with a contact stylus as quickly and as accurately as possible over a 30 s period. Contacts with either target (hits) or with the surrounding facia (misses) complete an electric circuit and register on digital counters. Four different target sizes were used (2 cm, 3 cm, 4 cm and 6 cm diameters). Targets were presented first in descending order and then in ascending order of size. A constant time interval of one minute was observed between each 30 s trial. The subject used the preferred hand. Two measures were analyzed from this task:

1) The number of total contacts (hits + misses) for each target size over each 30 s period.

2) The percentage of total contacts for each target size which missed the target. (These misses will be referred to as errors).

## 4 Analysis of Data

The results were analyzed using repeated measures analysis of variance. Where appropriate, paired comparisons were undertaken using correlated t-tests. For the Gibson spiral maze, the analyses of variance were run with two trial factors: treatment (lormetazepam; nitrazepam; and placebo); and test session (session 1 after the first dose and session 2 after the seventh dose). For the reciprocal tapping task the analyses of variance contained a further trial factor: target size (6 cm; 4 cm; 3 cm and 2 cm).

## 5 Results

None of the test measurements from the Gibson spiral maze showed significant main effects of, or significant interaction effects with, drug treatment.

For the reciprocal tapping task, total contacts showed no significant main effects of, and no significant interaction effects with, drug treatment. Analysis of percent errors, however, while showing no significant main effect of drug, did show two significant effects:

1) drug treatment × session ($F = 8.26$; $df = 2.22$; $p < 0.005$); and
2) drug treatment × target × session ($F = 2.85$; $df = 6.66$; $p < 0.05$).

The two-way interaction (drug treatment by session) is shown in Fig. 1. T-tests calculated between the drug treatment means for each session in turn showed that while neither lormetazepam nor nitrazepam differed significantly from placebo at session 1, performance associated with nitrazepam was significantly impaired at session 2 relative to both lormetazepam ($t = 2.54$; $df = 11$; $p < 0.05$) and placebo ($t = 3.00$; $df = 11$; $p < 0.01$; see Table 1).

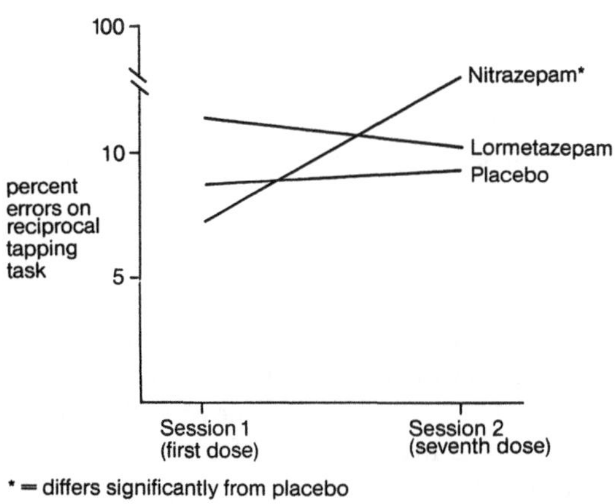


**Fig. 1.** Effects of nitrazepam, lormetazepam, and placebo on overall accuracy in reciprocal tapping. Drug treatment × session: $F = 8.26$; $df = 2.22$; $p < 0.005$

**Table 1.** Reciprocal tapping task (mean percent errors). Values of $t$ (correlated) for paired comparisons

| Treatment | | versus | Treatment | $t$-value | $p$[a] |
|---|---|---|---|---|---|
| *After a single dose* | | | | | |
| Lormetazepam | 1 mg | | Placebo | 1.45 | 0.175 |
| Nitrazepam | 5 mg | | Placebo | 0.63 | 0.543 |
| Lormetazepam | 1 mg | | Nitrazepam 5 mg | 2.90 | 0.014 |
| *After seven consecutive doses* | | | | | |
| Lormetazepam | 1 mg | | Placebo | 0.87 | 0.402 |
| Nitrazepam | 5 mg | | Placebo | 3.00 | 0.012 |
| Lormetazepam | 1 mg | | Nitrazepam 5 mg | 2.54 | 0.028 |

[a] Two-tailed significance values throughout

The significant three-way interaction (drug treatment by target × session) was further analyzed by repeating the analyses of variance for each target size. The 6 cm and 4 cm targets showed no significant main effect of, and no interaction effects with the drug factor. Both the 3 cm and the 2 cm target sizes, however, showed significant interactions between drug and test session ($F = 12.43$; $df = 2.22$; $p < 0.001$, for the 3 cm targets; and $F = 3.76$; $df = 2.22$; $p < 0.05$, for the 2 cm targets).

For the 3 cm targets paired comparisons between the drug treatments at each of the test sessions showed that, after single doses, neither lormetazepam nor nitrazepam differed from placebo. After seven consecutive doses, however, performance under nitrazepam was significantly worse than that associated with both placebo ($t = 3.46$; $df = 11$; $p < 0.01$), and lormetazepam($t = 3.32$; $df = 11$; $p < 0.01$). For the 2 cm targets, there were no significant differences between either of the drug treatments and placebo after a single dose, but significantly more errors were made following seven consecutive doses of both nitrazepam ($t = 2.32$; $df = 11$; $p < 0.05$) and lormetazepam ($t = 2.50$; $df = 11$; $p < 0.05$).

## 6 Conclusions

Task complexity on the reciprocal tapping test increases as the target sizes decrease. The figure shows that, irrespective of target size, nitrazepam was associated with an overall impairment after seven consecutive doses. That errors increased for nitrazepam between the first and seventh consecutive doses, but decreased for lormetazepam over the same period, suggests accumulation of nitrazepam. At low levels of task complexity (6 cm and 4 cm targets) neither drug was associated with impairment of performance.

At intermediate levels of task complexity (3 cm targets), nitrazepam showed a pattern of impairment similar to that shown in the figure, with errors increasing between the first and seventh dose of drug. Lormetazepam values for this target size, however, differ little from placebo. At the highest level of task complexity (2 cm targets) the pattern of performance decrements associated with nitrazepam remains consistent with a cumulative effect, again increasing between the first and the seventh doses. The performance decrement associated with lormetazepam for the 2 cm targets, however, was not consistent with a cumulative effect. For this target size, mean errors under the lormetazepam condition showed a decrease between the first and the seventh doses.

Neither drug significantly influenced the number of total contacts made in the reciprocal tapping test. This implies that the drug effects reported here do not result from an overall, non-specific, slowing of performance, but rather reflect a specific influence on the judgement and accuracy of the elderly subjects.

## References

Castleden CM, George CF, Marcer D, Hallett C (1977) Increased sensitivity to nitrazepam in old age. Br Med J 1:10–12

Gibson HB (1978) Manual to the Gibson spiral maze, 2nd edn. Hodder and Stoughton Educational, Sevenoaks, Kent

Morgan K (1982) Effect of low dose nitrazepam on performance in the elderly. Lancet 1:516

Salem SAM, Kinney CD, McDevitt DG (1982) Pharmacokinetics and psychomotor effects of nitrazepam and temazepam in healthy elderly males and females. Br J Clin Pharmacol 13(4):601–602

Pattie AH, Gilleard CJ (1975) A brief psychogeriatric assessment schedule. Br J Psychiatry 127:489–493

Swift CG, Haythorne JM, Clarke P, Stevenson IH (1981) The effect of ageing on measured responses to single doses of oral temazepam. Br J Clin Pharmacol 11:413–414

# Hypnotic Drugs for 1984

I. Oswald[1]

**Contents**



**Abstract**

It is still insufficiently recognised that hypnotics and anti-anxiety drugs are one and the same and that the regular intake of these drugs will be followed by withdrawal phenomena, including complaints of insomnia and anxiety. The long-acting, cumulative drugs like phenobarbitone or flurazepam cannot in reality be withdrawn abruptly owing to their persistence in the tissues, and so they do not cause sharp rebound phenomena, though they cause impaired skills and judgement by day.

Very short life drugs, like triazolam, are followed by immediate and severe withdrawal insomnia in older people and their regular nighttime intake may cause regular daytime withdrawal symptoms of enhanced anxiety. A hypnotic with a half-life of about 10 hours may be the most sensible compromise to provide sleep by night without serious positive or negative daytime effects, though some eventual withdrawal features will be inevitable. The benzodiazepines lead to a degree of tolerance, but this is never complete and their positive effects are sustained over many months.

Increased sleep duration has been assumed to be a necessary feature of an effective hypnotic. However, hypnotic drugs for the future might not lengthen sleep, but improve it's restorative value and the subjective satisfaction given to the patient.

**Key Words**

Alcohol/Anxiety/Chloral/Flurazepam/Fosazepam/Glutethimide/Loprazolam/Lormetazepam/ Methaqualone/Methyprylone/Nitrazepam/Paraldehyde/Protein synthesis/Tolerance/Trazodone/Urinary cortisol/Visual analogue scales/Withdrawal rebound phenomena.

1 University Department of Psychiatry, Royal Edinburgh Hospital, GB-Edinburgh, EH10 5HF

Psychopharmacology Supplementum 1
Editors: I. Hindmarch, H. Ott and T. Roth

# 1 Introduction

Among the issues we must consider is whether a hypnotic drug should be cumulative and lead to daytime dopiness, or whether it should be short-acting and possibly even lead to daytime withdrawal symptoms. Then too we must think about the nature of withdrawal rebound phenomena; also the importance of age as a determinant of brain sensitivity to a drug, as well as how age may affect its elimination; also the degree to which effects of a benzodiazepine may be sustained over many months; and whether hypnotics of the more distant future have functions other than the mere prolongation of sleep.

# 2 Withdrawal Syndrome

## 2.1 Safety Aspect

Recent years have seen large numbers of patients admitted to hospitals around the world on account of overdoses of drugs and a feature of recent years in Edinburgh has been the steadily falling proportion of such patients who are admitted unconscious. Credit must go to the benzodiazepines, which are very safe, and so they will continue to have advantage.

## 2.2 Dose Dependency

Administration of a benzodiazepine derivative soothes anxiety and promotes sleep. During continued use, the brain adjusts to the drug, becoming modified to counteract the drug's action, and we observe tolerance in some degree. Then if the drug is suddenly withdrawn, the new modifications remain in the brain and bring about the opposite of the drug's effects, namely enhanced anxiety, diminished sleep, and usually an enhanced proportion of REM sleep. It is sometimes asked how long a drug must be taken before these rebound withdrawal effects can be seen and the answer must be that it depends on the dose. A single very large dose, taken by someone not previously on drugs, will produce initial positive effects and then rebound withdrawal phenomena, so that in former times delirium was not uncommon a few days after an overdose of some of the barbiturates, methaqualone or methyprylone (Haider and Oswald 1970). It is impossible abruptly to withdraw drugs like phenobarbitone or flurazepam, owing to the long persistence in the body of active substance, and so withdrawal rebound phenomena are not easily seen (Kales et al. 1982) unless the drug has been taken in overdose, when the rebound may be seen after either of these drugs (Haider and Oswald 1970; Oswald 1980a).

## 2.3 Drug Characteristics

The withdrawal syndrome of anxiety and insomnia after a hypnotic has been recognised for centuries in the case of alcohol, for a hundred years in the case of paraldehyde and was well described for other drugs such as chloral, glutethimide and the barbiturates (Wulff 1959). Rebound phenomena were recognised from the early days of benzodiazepines (Oswald and Priest 1965) and particularly insomnia after nitrazepam (Adam et al. 1976), while Petursson and Lader (1981) have reported many of the other features, especially anxiety. The immediacy with which rebound phenomena reach their peak depends upon how rapidly the drug leaves the brain (Oswald 1973) and sometimes EEG studies of sleep can be a more useful guide than plasma half-life studies. Some years ago we studied fosazepam, at a time when the primary compound was believed to have a half-life of about three hours. We found in our sleep studies that some of the withdrawal features peaked on the fourth night and predicted that longer life products would be discovered, as was indeed soon found to be the case (Allen and Oswald 1976). More recently we have conducted studies of loprazolam, finding that withdrawal effects peaked on the third night after stopping the drug. We had been informed by the pharmaceutical company that loprazolam had a six-hour half-life, but are not surprised that the half-life has now been reported to be sixteen hours (Jochemsen 1983).

## 2.4 Patient Differentiation

It was Castleden et al. (1977) who proposed that the brain of elderly people is more sensitive to a given concentration of a benzodiazepine, though, of course, it must be remembered that the liver may function less effectively and drugs may be eliminated more slowly in the elderly.

Whereas young people may be little impaired by a regular intake of nitrazepam 5 mg nightly, a woman of 88, in generally good health, may become progressively more inert and become subject to falls if she regularly takes the same dose, simply because higher tissue levels accumulate.

Older people have more broken sleep under natural circumstances and it is not surprising perhaps that they may be more severely affected by drug withdrawal. Many young people sleep so well that it is difficult either to improve or to impair their sleep. In San Diego, Spinweber and Johnson (1982) gave triazolam 0.5 mg nightly to ten young men aged about 21 for six consecutive nights. On withdrawal their sleep differed little from baseline circumstances. It is true that there were only six nights on active drug and that baseline nights may have been somewhat disturbed by insufficient adaptation to the laboratory, but the apparent lack of any withdrawal rebound was in sharp contrast to our recent experience in Edinburgh when nine poor sleepers, of mean age 61 years, received triazolam 0.5 mg nightly for twenty-one nights. In comparison with earlier baseline nights, when triazolam was withdrawn and placebos substituted, there was severe insomnia, most marked on the first withdrawal night, when total sleep averaged only 255 min, compared with a baseline mean of 446 min. Similarly, overnight urinary cortisol shot up to significantly higher levels on the first withdrawal night (Adam et al. 1984). The important difference from the San Diego study must have been those additional forty years of age.

## 2.5 Daytime Anxiety

All hypnotic drugs are anti-anxiety drugs, so that withdrawal is associated with a sense of unease. If we think for a moment of someone who takes the traditional anti-anxiety drug, alcohol, which is metabolised within a few hours, and if, let us suppose, he is someone who confines his drinking to a bottle of gin regularly each evening, then we shall not be surprised if he wakens in the morning feeling tense and anxious and even more certainly feels tense and anxious during the day until he gets relief from his evening bottle and then sleeps. Triazolam is a much safer drug, but it also is very rapidly metabolised and a dose of 0.5 mg nightly is twice the maximum recommended British dose, indeed four times the recommended British dose for older people (though as much as 1 mg is in use in some European countries and 0.5 mg in the U.S.A.). When my colleagues and I gave 21 poor sleepers of late middle age loprazolam 1 mg nightly for three weeks, they became significantly less anxious compared with a prior baseline week on placebos (an adaptation week on placebos having preceded this too). They rated their daytime anxiety by filling in visual analogue scales each evening. When the same people, some before and some after the loprazolam experience, took triazolam 0.5 mg nightly for three weeks, they became on average steadily more anxious, significantly so by the third week, as shown in their analogue ratings (Morgan and Oswald 1982). I am sure that the fact that they had a mean age of 56 years was important, in relation to the large dose used and that had a more modest dose been taken, then no significant anxiety effect would have emerged.

## 3 Experience and Outlook

### 3.1 Previous Studies

Doctors often ask whether the benzodiazepines become ineffective with continued intake. To some degree there is tolerance, as with other hypnotics, but the

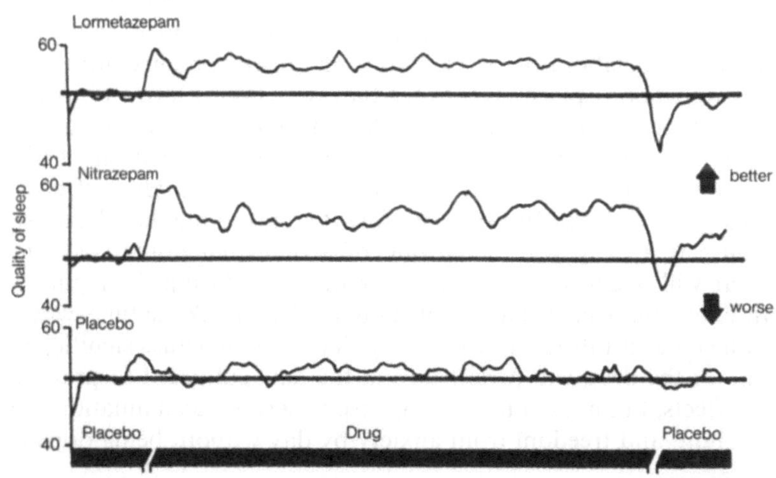


**Fig. 1.** Daily self-ratings of quality of sleep during 32 weeks, smoothed and shown as five-point moving means. Compared with placebo, both drugs appeared to cause sustained improvement during the period of active treatment, with rebound worsening after withdrawal. (Horizontal lines represent baseline means). Reproduced with permission from the British Medical Journal (Oswald et al. 1982)

degree of tolerance is never complete. At Edinburgh we entered 100 selected poor sleepers of late middle age into a study in which each participated for 32 weeks, taking capsules each night and making a variety of self-ratings daily. Twenty-five received placebos throughout, and twenty-five received placebos for the first four weeks, then nitrazepam for 24 weeks, then placebos again for four weeks. Fifty received lormetazepam 2 mg nightly during the middle twenty-four weeks, preceded and followed by placebos. Among the interesting findings that emerged was a small but significant fall in body weight in both the benzodiazepine groups, whereas the placebo group did not change in weight at all (Oswald and Adam 1980). It reminds us that there is much we do not know about the benzodiazepines. Among the self-ratings was an estimate each morning of what had been the sleep latency, and a judgement of the quality of sleep. Steady intake of placebos during 32 weeks had no effect on either of these measures. As soon as the subject started on either of the benzodiazepines there was a significant improvement in sleep latency and in sleep quality and inspection of Fig. 1 confirms that there was a sustained effect from both the active drugs, with a sharp impairment caused by withdrawal rebound effects as an inevitable corollary of some prior tolerance, but that does not diminish the importance of the sustained positive effect.

### 3.2 Optimum Benzodiazepine

Which is the optimum benzodiazepine hypnotic? There is a wide choice. One may choose a long-life benzodiazepine that is cumulative in its action like flurazepam. Because abrupt withdrawal is impossible, there will be no sharp let-down if the drug is stopped and the drug will persist in its actions, in diminishing degree, for several nights. My colleagues and I are among those who have found impressive daytime impairment in middle-aged people taking flurazepam 30 mg nightly for three weeks. Particularly serious was the high rate of social and general life disasters outside the testing laboratory while they took flurazepam, in contrast to the time when they were taking placebos or when they were taking lormetazepam. (Oswald et al. 1979). I regard flurazepam as obsolete, in characteristics much like phenobarbitone. At the other end of the scale there is the extremely short-life triazolam, and I have already referred to the consequent disadvantages of daytime rebound anxiety. At the present time therefore it seems to me that the most sensible compromise is a drug with a half-life of around ten hours, such as lormetazepam, that will reach high enough concentrations during the night to ensure a hypnotic effect, but which will be half eliminated by breakfast time, when the remaining tissue concentrations may not be high enough to cause significant impairment. Some of the drug will persist during the day, sufficient to prevent daytime rebound effects, but not enough to give rise to serious accumulation, so ensuring sleep at night, and freedom from anxiety by day without being doped.

### 3.3 Future Hypnotics and Therapeutic Criteria

Turning to prophecy and speculation, what might be sought for hypnotics of the future? There is a general belief that sleep is restorative and today we have available a wealth of evidence that there are major differences across the 24 hours in the rate of renewal of body tissues, the highest rate of protein synthesis in, for example, the brain, coinciding with the sleep period (Danait and Rebiere 1978). How hypnotic drugs affect such functions we do not know, and to find out must remain a challenge for future research. Those of us who have worked with the EEG to study sleep must realise that we should not be too preoccupied with it, for it tells us nothing about sleep's restorative properties. We can recognise that subjective opinion is highly important as an indicator of whether or not a hypnotic will succeed commercially. In recent studies at Edinburgh, we have examined the effects of trazodone 150 mg nightly on the sleep of middle-aged poor sleepers. It is sold as an anti-depressant drug, but our subjects rated their sleep significantly improved in quality. Yet there was no significant effect on sleep latency or on sleep duration. What was remarkable was a great increase in time spent in slow-wave sleep, stages 3 and 4 (Montgomery et al. 1984). These latter stages have often been regarded as in some way worth more (Dement and Greenberg 1966; Oswald 1980b). It is just possible that there is a connection between the greater amount of slow-wave sleep and the subjective opinion of improved quality of sleep in the absence of altered sleep duration. My reason for mentioning these experimental findings is to suggest that the search for a drug that increases sleep duration may not be the only path for the future. In theory one might think there could exist a drug that would shorten sleep, yet so improve its quality and restorative properties, that people would feel that they had a better night's sleep and also be able to ply their intellectual and social skills by day to highest standards.

## References

Adam K, Adamson L, Březinová V, Hunter WM, Oswald I (1976) Nitrazepam: lastingly effective but trouble on withdrawal. Br Med J 1:1558–1560

Adam K, Oswald I, Shapiro C (1984) Effects of loprazolam and of triazolam on sleep and overnight urinary cortisol. (To be published)

Allen S, Oswald I (1976) Anxiety and sleep after fosazepam. Br J Clin Pharmacol 3:165–168

Castleden CM, George CF, Marcer D, Hallett C (1977) Increased sensitivity to nitrazepam in old age. Br Med J 1:10–12

Danait J, Rebiere A (1978) Daily variations of the in vivo ($^3$H) leucine incorporation into the cerebellar and cerebral proteins of the normal and hypothyroid young rat. Experientia (Basel) 34:264–265

Dement W, Greenberg S (1966) Changes in total amount of stage four sleep as a function of partial sleep deprivation. Electroenceph Clin Neurophysiol 20:523–526

Haider I, Oswald I (1970) Late brain recovery processes after drug overdose. Br Med J 2:318–322

Jochemsen R (1983) Clinical pharmacokinetics of benzodiazepine hypnotics. Drukkerij JH Pasmans BV, 's-Gravenhage

Kales A, Bixler EO, Soldatos CR, Vela-Bueno A, Jacoby J, Kales JD (1982) Quazepam and flurazepam: long-term use and extended withdrawal. Clin Pharmacol Ther 32:781–788

Montgomery I, Oswald I, Morgan K, Adam K (1984) Trazodone enhances sleep in subjective quality but not in objective duration. Br J Clin Pharmacol (in press)

Morgan K, Oswald I (1982) Anxiety caused by a short-life hypnotic. Br Med J 284:942

Oswald I (1973) Drug research and human sleep. Annu Rev Pharmacol 53:243–252

Oswald I (1980a) Sleep studies in clinical pharmacology. Br J Clin Pharmacol 10:317–326

Oswald I (1980b) Sleep as a restorative process: Human clues. Prog Brain Res 53:279–288

Oswald I, Priest RG (1965) Five weeks to escape the sleeping-pill habit. Br Med J 2:1093–1099
Oswald I, Adam K, Borrow S, Idzikowski C (1979) The effects of two hypnotics on sleep, subjective feeling and skilled performance. In: Passouant P, Oswald I (eds) Pharmacology of the states of alertness. Pergamon Press, Oxford, pp 51–63
Oswald I, Adam K (1980) Benzodiazepines cause small loss of body weight. Br Med J 281:1039–1040
Oswald I, French C, Adam K, Gilham J (1982) Benzodiazepine hypnotics remain effective for 24 weeks. Br Med J 284:860–863
Petursson H, Lader MH (1981) Withdrawal from long-term benzodiazepine treatment. Br Med J 283:643–645
Spinweber CL, Johnson LC (1982) Effects of triazolam (0.5 mg) on sleep, performance, memory and arousal threshold. Psychopharmacology (Berlin) 76:5–12
Wulff MH (1959) The barbiturate withdrawal syndrome. Electroencephalogr Clin Neurophysiol [Suppl] 14:1–161

# Pharmacokinetics and Pharmacodynamics of Benzodiazepines

# Pharmacodynamics of Benzodiazepines After Single Oral Doses: Kinetic and Physiochemical Correlates

D. J. Greenblatt[1], R. M. Arendt[2] and R. I. Shader[1]

**Contents**



**Abstract**

Differences among various benzodiazepines in onset and intensity of action after single oral doses are not attributable to differences in blood brain barrier permeability. When given parenterally all benzodiazepines rapidly enter brain tissue and have a rapid onset of action, indicating that passage from blood to brain is not the rate-limiting factor (Arendt et al. 1983). Rather it is the difference in rate of absorption – passage from the gastrointestinal tract to systemic blood – that largely determines the onset of action after single oral doses. This difference in absorption rate in turn depends on the relative lipophilicity as well as the characteristics of the pharmaceutical formulation. There are benefits and disadvantages associated with rapid as well as with slow absorption profiles, depending on the clinical situation and the patient's expectations and particular pattern of drug sensitivity. The suggestion that a drug "works promptly but does not produce initial euphoria" is contradictory, since rapid absorption is the mechanism for both of these effects.

**Key Words**

Abusability/Absorption rate/Alprazolam/Brotizolam/Chlordiazepoxide/Clobazam/Desalkylflurazepam/Desmethyldiazepam/Diazepam/Flunitrazepam/Lorazepam/Midazolam/Oxazepam/Pharmaceutical formulation/Prazepam/Physiochemical characteristics/Temazepam/Triazolam.

## 1 Introduction

Comparisons of antianxiety efficacy among various benzodiazepines during short or intermediate duration treatment of neurotic anxiety generally demonstrate that appropriately chosen doses of any benzodiazepine are similar in efficacy to each other and more effective than placebo (Greenblatt and Shader 1974, 1978; Rickels 1978). Most of these clinical comparisons focus on drug efficacy during

1 Division of Clinical Pharmacology, Department of Psychiatry and Medicine, Tufts-New England Medical Center, Boston, MA 02111, USA
2 Institute of Anesthesiology, Medizinische Universitätsklinik, University of Bonn, D-5300 Bonn, FRG

Psychopharmacology Supplementum 1
Editors: I. Hindmarch, H. Ott and T. Roth

repeated use, with the usual trial duration ranging from one to four weeks. Recent evidence suggests that the clinical similarity during repeated administration might not apply to the single-dosing situation. Large differences appear to exist among the benzodiazepine derivatives in the onset, intensity and duration of their clinical actions after single oral doses in humans (Kanto 1981; Johnson and Chernik 1982; Wittenborn 1979; Kothary et al. 1981). Such differences assume potentially great importance when one evaluates the use of benzodiazepines for therapeutic purposes in single-dose "p.r.n." situations during treatment of anxiety or insomnia, or when the profile of side effects or abuse potential of the various compound is compared.

## 2 The Importance of Absorption Rate

The time of onset and intensity of action of benzodiazepines after single oral doses appear to depend on the rate of absorption from the gastrointestinal tract (Greenblatt et al. 1983; Bliding 1974). Benzodiazepines with rapid rates of absorption rapidly cross the lipoidal barriers of the gastrointestinal tract mucosa, enter the portal circulation, and thereafter enter the systemic circulation. Under these circumstances, human subjects or patients will perceive rapid onset of clinical effects that are increasingly intense depending on the size of the dose. The rapid and intense onset of single-dose effects may be favourable or unfavourable depending on the clinical situation. Patients who link therapeutic benefit to this prompt pharmacologic effect perceive it as therapeutically beneficial. Fast absorption also is important when benzodiazepines are used for the treatment of insomnia in individuals whose sleep disorder is characterized mainly by difficulty falling asleep ("sleep-latency insomnia"). Some patients, however, may perceive the intense single-dose effect as dysphoric, being associated with a feeling of drowsiness, excessive relaxation, feeling "spaced out", or loss of control. It is further suggested, but not proven, that the reinforcing effects of rapidly absorbed benzodiazepines such as diazepam and clorazepate may increase their "abusability", in that persons using these drugs for pleasure-seeking rather than therapeutic purposes may select those drugs that are most rapidly absorbed and most promptly reinforcing (Stitzer et al. 1981; Griffiths and Ator 1981).

The converse clinical profile can be anticipated for benzodiazepines that are slowly absorbed from the gastrointestinal tract (Bliding 1974). Since oral doses slowly reach the systemic circulation, the onset of single-dose effects are slower and of reduced intensity. Such drugs may be unfavourable for patients with sleep-latency insomnia or those who require prompt onset of effects to alleviate acute or anticipatory anxiety. On the other hand, slow absorption may be a favourable property for those who wish to avoid the drowsy or "spaced out" feeling that they may experience when absorption is rapid.

Clinicians utilizing benzodiazepines in clinical practice have some degree of control on the rate of drug absorption. Benzodiazepines as well as other drugs generally are more rapidly absorbed when taken in the fasting state. Drug absorption can be slowed by administering the agents on a full stomach (Greenblatt et al. 1978; Divoll et al. 1982) with aluminum-containing antacids (Greenblatt et al.

1976, 1978; Shader et al. 1978), or by coadministration of other agents that may reduce gastrointestinal motility and thereby slowing the rate of gastric emptying. Controlled studies suggest that for any given benzodiazepine in any given individual, slowing of the rate of absorption by coadministration of an aluminum antacid significantly reduces the subjective perception of the onset and intensity of the effects (Shader et al. 1978; Greenblatt et al. 1977).

Although circumstances of administration partly influence benzodiazepine absorption rate, most of the variability in absorption rate is determined by intrinsic physiochemical characteristics of the various benzodiazepines, together with the characteristics of the pharmaceutical formulation. Table 1 summarizes findings from studies of healthy young individuals who ingested single oral therapeutic doses of various benzodiazepines with 100–200 ml of tap water after an overnight fast. The time of peak concentration of each drug was determined by measurement of drug concentrations in plasma at multiple time points following the single dose. The table demonstrates great differences among the various drugs in the time of peak concentration, despite controlled circumstances of administration in a homogenous study population. Diazepam is the most rapidly absorbed benzodiazepine, with peak concentrations reaching an average of 0.88 hours after dosage. The next most rapidly absorbed is desmethyldiazepam administered as the precursor clorazepate, with peak levels at 1.18 hours after the dose. At the other end of the spectrum is desmethyldiazepam formed from its precursor prazepam, which does not peak until 7.8 hours. Other benzodiazepines fall between these extremes. The pharmaceutical formulation clearly contributes to

**Table 1.** Time of peak plasma concentration following single oral doses of various benzodiazepines administered to healthy young volunteers in the fasting state

| Drug | Dosage Form[a] | Time of peak concentration [h] | |
|---|---|---|---|
| | | Mean | Range |
| Diazepam | Tablet (Valium, Roche) | 0.88 | (0.08–2.5) |
| Clorazepate (yielding DMDZ) | Capsule (Tranxene, Abbott) | 1.18 | (0.5–2.5) |
| Alprazolam | Tablet (Xanax, Upjohn) | 1.40 | (0.25–4.0) |
| Triazolam | Tablet (Halcion, Upjohn) | 1.80 | (0.5–6.0) |
| Lorazepam | Tablet (Ativan, Wyeth) | 1.88 | (0.5–6.0) |
| Oxazepam | Tablet (Serax, Wyeth) | 2.31 | (0.5–6.0) |
| Temazepam | Capsule (Restoril, Sandoz) | 2.46 | (0.75–4.0) |
| Prazepam (yielding DMDZ) | Tablet (Verstran, Warner-Lambert) | 7.8 | (2.5–24.0) |

[a] American trade name and manufacturer shown in parenthesis

some of these differences. For example, the hard capsule preparation of temazepam available in the United States (Restoril®, Sandoz) is much more slowly absorbed than is the soft gelatine capsule available in the United Kingdom (Divoll et al. 1981; Fuccella et al. 1977). The clinical consequences of these formulation differences are evident in controlled studies which indicate that the American capsule preparation of temazepam has inconsistent efficacy in the treatment of insomnia characterized primarily by difficulty in falling asleep (Mitler 1981).

## 3 Mechanism of Differences in Absorption Rate

Differences among benzodiazepines in lipophilicity or lipid-solubility have recently received attention as a possible physiochemical explanation for their differing rates of absorption. At present it is not established which, if any, in vitro index of lipid solubility relates best to drug behaviour in vivo. One traditional approach to evaluating lipid solubility utilizes the properties of a drug's partitioning at equilibrium between an aqueous medium and an organic solvent (Chiou et al. 1981; Leo et al. 1971). Of many variants of this approach, the octanol:buffer partition ratio is utilized extensively. Increasing lipophilicity is associated with greater partitioning into organic as opposed to aqueous phases after equilibrium is attained. Figure 1 shows data on the octanol:buffer partition ratios for various benzodiazepines at physiologic pH (Greenblatt et al. in press). All benzodiazepines are highly lipid-soluble, having partition ratios considerably larger than unity. Nonetheless the drugs differ among themselves in lipophilicity. Diazepam

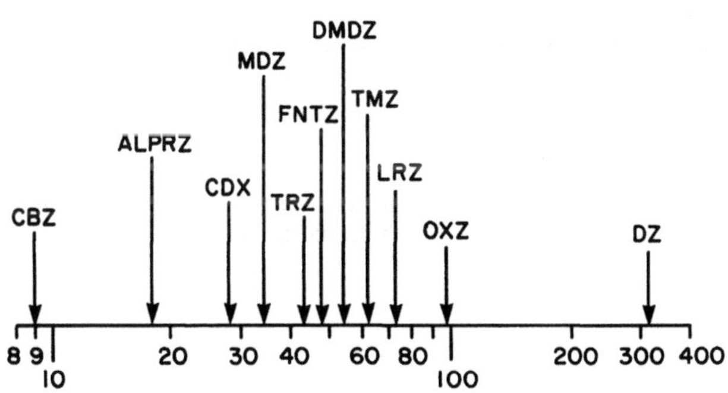


**Fig. 1.** Octanol:buffer partition coefficients of various benzodiazepines (see list of abbreviations)

| *List of Abbreviations* | | | | | |
|---|---|---|---|---|---|
| | | LRZ | Lorazepam | MDZ | Midazolam |
| | | TMZ | Temazepam | CDX | Chlordiazepoxide |
| DZ | Diazepam | FNTZ | Flunitrazepam | CBZ | Clobazam |
| DMDZ | Desmethyldiazepam | TRZ | Triazolam | BTZ | Brotizolam |
| OXZ | Oxazepam | ALPRZ | Alprazolam | DAFLZ | Desalkylflurazepam |

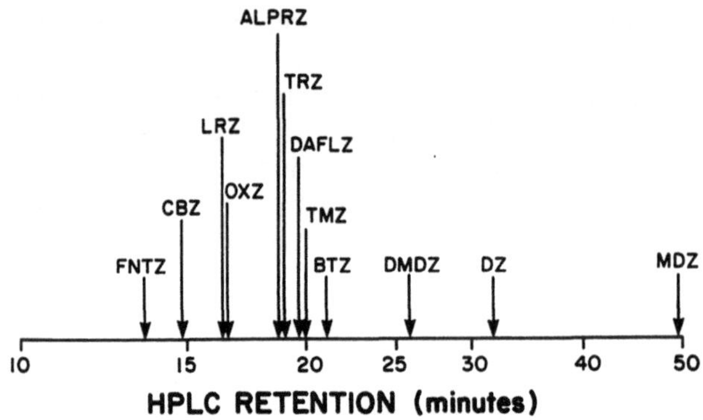


**Fig. 2.** High pressure liquid chromatographic (HPLC) retention times of various benzodiazepines (see list of abbreviations)

is the most lipid soluble of benzodiazepines, consistent with its rapid absorption rate (Ochs et al. 1982), but the scheme has some important inconsistencies. For example, oxazepam has a relatively high partition ratio but a slow rate of absorption in vivo, whereas desmethyldiazepam has a lower partition ratio but a much more rapid absorption rate than oxazepam. In our laboratory we have evaluated liquid chromatographic retention as another approach to assessing lipophilicity (Greenblatt et al. in press). Retention time on a reverse-phase high pressure liquid chromatographic (HPLC) system for any given compound is known to depend in part on its polarity, with more lipophilicity compounds retained longest (Hulshoff and Perrin 1976; Butte et al. 1981; Smith and Jungalwala 1981). Retention times of the various benzodiazepines were determined using a reverse-phase C-18 chromatographic column at physiologic pH and at a fixed flow rate. Figure 2 again demonstrates that all benzodiazepines are lipophilic, but differ among themselves in lipophilicity. Midazolam, diazepam and desmethyldiazepam have prolonged retention due to their high lipid solubility, whereas hydroxylated benzodiazepines such as oxazepam and lorazepam have a much shorter retention. The HPLC retention index appears to relate more closely to in vivo characteristics of distribution and rate of absorption than does octanol:buffer partitioning (Greenblatt et al. in press; Arendt et al. 1983).

*Acknowledgements.* We are grateful for the collaboration and assistance of Dr. Darrell R. Abernethy, Dr. Hermann R. Ochs, Ann Locniskar, and Jerold S. Harmatz.

## References

Arendt RM, Greenblatt DJ, DeJong RH, Abernethy DR, Sellers EM (1983) Benzodiazepine entry into CSF and brain: Kinetic, dynamic, and in vitro correlations. Clin Pharmacol Ther 33:239

Bliding A (1974) Effects of different rates of absorption of two benzodiazepines on subjective and objective parameters. Eur J Clin Pharmocol 7:201–211

Butte W, Fooken C, Klussman R, Schuller D (1981) Evaluation of lipophilic properties for a series of phenols, using reversed-phase high-performance liquid chromatography and high-performance thin-layer chromatography. J Chromatogr 214:59–67

Chiou CT, Schmedding DW, Block JH (1981) Correlation of water solubility with octanol-water partition coefficient. J Pharm Sci 70:1176–1177

Divoll M, Greenblatt DJ, Harmatz JS, Shader RI (1981) Effect of age and gender on disposition of temazepam. J Pharm Sci 70:1104–1107
Divoll M, Greenblatt DJ, Ciraulo DA, Puri SK, Ho I, Shader RI (1982) Clobazam kinetics: Intra-subject variability, and effect of food on absorption. J Clin Pharmacol 22:69–73
Fuccella LM, Bolcioni G, Tamassia V, Ferrario L, Tognoni G (1977) Human pharmacokinetics and bioavailability of temazepam administered in soft gelatin capsules. Eur J Clin Pharmacol 12:383–386
Greenblatt DJ, Shader RI (1974) Benzodiazepines in clinical practice. Raven Press, New York
Greenblatt DJ, Shader RI, Harmatz JS, Franke K, Koch-Weser J (1976) Influence on magnesium and aluminum hydroxide mixture on chlordiazepoxide absorption. Clin Pharmacol Ther 19:234–239
Greenblatt DJ, Shader RI, Harmatz JS, Franke K, Koch-Weser J (1977) Absorption rate, blood concentrations, and early response to oral chlordiazepoxide. Am J Psychiatry 134:559–562
Greenblatt DJ, Shader RI (1978) Pharmacotherapy of anxiety with benzodiazepines and β-adrenergic blockers. In: Lipton MA, DiMascio A, Killiam KF (eds) Psychopharmacology: A generation of progress. Raven Press, New York, pp 1381-1389
Greenblatt DJ, Allen MD, MacLaughlin DS, Harmatz JS, Shader RI (1978) Diazepam absorption: Effect of antacids and food. Clin Pharmacol Ther 24:600–609
Greenblatt DJ, Divoll M, Abernethy DR, Ochs HR, Shader RI (1983) Benzodiazepine kinetics: Implications for therapeutics and pharmacogeriatrics. Drug Metab Rev 14:251–292
Greenblatt DJ, Arendt RM, Abernethy DR, Giles HG, Sellers EM, Shader RI (1984). In vitro quantitation of benzodiazepine lipophilicity: Relation to in vivo distribution. Br J Anaesth (in press)
Griffiths RR, Ator NA (1981) Benzodiazepine self-administration in animals and humans: A comprehensive literature review. In: Szara SI, Ludford JP (eds) (1980) Benzodiazepines: A review of research results (NIDA Research Monograph No. 33, DHHS Publication No. (ADM) 81-1052). Government Printing Office, Washington, DC
Hulshoff A, Perrin JH (1976) A comparison of the determination of partition coefficients of 1,4-benzodiazepines by high-performance liquid chromatography and thin-layer chromatography. J Chromatogr 129:263–276
Johnson LC, Chernik DA (1982) Sedative-hypnotics and human performance. Psychopharmacology (Berlin) 76:101–113
Kanto J (1981) Benzodiazepines as oral premedicants. Br J Anaesth 53:1179–1188
Kothary SP, Brown ACD, Pandit UA, Samra SK, Pandit SK (1981) Time course of antirecall effect of diazepam and lorazepam following oral administration. Anaesthesiol 55:641–644
Leo A, Hansch C, Elkins D (1971) Partition coefficients and their uses. Chem Rev 71:525–616
Mitler MM (1981) Evaluation of temazepam as a hypnotic. Pharmacother 1:3–11
Ochs HR, Otten H, Greenblatt DJ, Dengler JH (1982) Diazepam absorption: Effects of age, sex, and Billroth gastrectomy. Dig Dis Sci 27:740–744
Rickels K (1978) Use of antianxiety agents in anxious outpatients. Psychopharmacology (Berlin) 58:1–17
Shader RI, Georgotas A, Greenblatt DJ, Harmatz JS, Allen MD (1978) Impaired absorption of desmethyldiazepam from clorazepate by magnesium aluminum hydroxide. Clin Pharmacol Ther 24:308–315
Smith M, Jungalwala FB (1981) Reversed-phase high performance liquid chromatography of phosphatidylcholine: A simple method for determining relative hydrophobic interaction of various molecular species. J Lipid Res 22:697–704
Stitzer ML, Griffiths RR, McLellan AT, Grabowski J, Hawthorne JW (1981) Diazepam use among methadone maintenance patients: Patterns and dosages. Drug Alcohol Depend 8:189–199
Wittenborn JR (1979) Effects of benzodiazepines on psychomotor performance. Br J Clin Pharmacol 7:S61–S67

# Lormetazepam – Plasma Concentrations in Volunteers Following Sublingual and Oral Dosing

D. K. Luscombe[1]

**Contents**



**Abstract**

The plasma profile of lormetazepam has been determined in sixteen clinically healthy, adult male volunteers following 1 mg lormetazepam, administered either sublingually or by the oral route.

Absorption of lormetazepam was found to be rapid following both sublingual and oral administration. While a trend was observed towards a more rapid rate of absorption after sublingual dosing, statistically, there was no significant difference ($p > 0.05$) between the speed with which lormetazepam was absorbed following sublingual and oral dosing.

After absorption, plasma lormetazepam levels rapidly reached mean ($\pm$ s.d.) peak concentrations of $4.9 \pm 0.9$ ng/ml and $5.2 \pm 1.7$ ng/ml for the sublingual and oral routes, respectively, there being no significant difference ($p > 0.05$) between these values. Likewise, there was no significant difference ($p > 0.05$) in the times at which peak plasma levels were attained in the two groups. Furthermore, measurement of the area under each plasma concentration-time curve showed that the bioavailability of lormetazepam was the same for the two routes of administration. Elimination of lormetazepam followed a similar pattern following sublingual and oral dosing, the mean terminal half-lives being 13.0 h and 13.8 h, respectively.

The findings in the present study clearly indicate that the plasma profiles of lormetazepam attained on sublingual and oral dosing are similar, indeed the pharmacokinetic characteristics of this drug appear identical being independent of its route of administration.

**Key Words**

Absorption/Bioavailability/Buccal cavity/Elimination/First-pass metabolism/Gastrointestinal tract/Pharmacokinetic characteristics/Plasma elimination/Plasma profile/Route of administration/Short-acting hypnotic.

1 Division of Applied Pharmacology, Welsh School of Pharmacy, UMIST, GB-Cardiff CF1 3MU

Psychopharmacology Supplementum 1
Editors: I. Hindmarch, H. Ott and T. Roth

# 1 Introduction

Lormetazepam is a benzodiazepine derivative with potent hypnotic activity (Heidrich et al. 1981). Following oral administration, rapid and complete absorption takes place (Hümpel et al. 1979) sleep being induced within 20 minutes of dosing (Oswald et al. 1978). While lormetazepam is effective for approximately six to eight hours (Oswald et al. 1978; Jovanovic et al. 1980) it exhibits no hangover effects the next morning (Heidrich et al. 1981).

Many of the patients who seek drug treatment for their insomnia find difficulty in swallowing oral dosage forms such as tablets and capsules. This is particularly so in the elderly. For this reason, a pharmacokinetic study has been carried out in volunteers to establish whether the sublingual route is suitable for the administration of lormetazepam. The aim of the study was therefore to determine the basic pharmacokinetic profile of lormetazepam in volunteers following oral dosing with 1 mg lormetazepam and to compare this profile with that achieved following sublingual dosing with 1 mg lormetazepam using the same dosage form (tablet) for both routes of administration.

# 2 Method

## 2.1 Volunteers

Sixteen clinically healthy, young, male subjects, who had not received a benzodiazepine or other form of medication for at least one week prior to the study, were selected for the study. Subjects were instructed not to take any other drug during the course of the study. The study was conducted with local Ethical Committee approval and with the informed consent of the volunteers.

## 2.2 Study Design

Following a light breakfast each volunteer was randomly assigned to either sublingual or oral dosage group. Volunteers receiving lormetazepam by the sublingual route were instructed to place a tablet under the tongue, to leave it stationary, and to limit swallowing to a minimum. These subjects reported the time at which the tablet had completely dispersed from under the tongue and this was found to be between 2 and 5 min. No fluid intake was permitted for the first 60 min of the study. Subjects taking the drug orally swallowed the preparation with half a glass of water, no further intake being permitted in the following hour. The dosage form in both instances was identical being a single Noctamid® tablet containing 1 mg lormetazepam.

## 2.3 Blood Collections

Venous blood samples (10 ml) were collected at time zero, 5, 10, 15, 30, 45, 60, 90 min, 2, 3, 4, 5, 7, 12, 24 and 30 h post-dosing. Blood was placed in lithium heparinized tubes and centrifuged. The plasma fraction was immediately separated and kept frozen at − 20 °C until required for analysis. Plasma concentrations of lormetazepam were determined using a specific radioreceptor assay procedure (Dorow et al. 1982).

## 3 Results

The mean (± s.d.) weight and age of volunteers in the sublingual group was 66.1 ± 6.2 kg and 26.1 ± 3.6 years, while the corresponding value in the oral group was 72.3 ± 9.0 kg and 24.9 ± 2.3 years, respectively. Statistically there was no significant difference ($p > 0.05$) between the two groups for each of these physiological parameters.

Lormetazepam was detected in the plasma of all volunteers following sublingual and oral dosing with 1 mg Noctamid®. Mean plasma concentrations for both groups are presented in Table 1 where it may be observed that lormetazepam was detectable within 10 min of sublingual dosing compared with 15 min for the oral route. Interestingly, while only two subjects in the oral group exhibited detectable plasma lormetazepam levels at 15 min, lormetazepam was present in the plasma of seven of the eight volunteers in the sublingual group after this time interval. Therefore, not only is lormetazepam capable of being absorbed sublingually but its rate of absorption certainly appears more rapid (Fig 1) than achieved after oral dosing. However, on subjecting the plasma data to statistical examination, the apparent trend of a more rapid rate of absorption could not be substantiated. Comparison of the mean values for the sublingual and oral groups at all time intervals up to 45 minutes post dosing, using Student's 't' test, indicated no significant difference ($p > 0.05$) in the speed with which lormetazepam appears in the plasma of the two groups.

**Table 1.** Mean plasma concentration of lormetazepam (ng/ml) in groups of 8 male volunteers who received 1 mg lormetazepam administered either sublingually or orally

| Time | Sublingual (mean ± s.d.) | Oral (mean ± s.d.) |
|---|---|---|
| 0 | 0 | 0 |
| 5 min | 0 | 0 |
| 10 min | 0.14 ± 0.07 | 0 |
| 15 min | 0.65 ± 0.14 | 0.06 ± 0.04 |
| 30 min | 1.93 ± 0.36 | 0.85 ± 0.35 |
| 45 min | 3.20 ± 0.60 | 2.69 ± 0.83 |
| 60 min | 3.54 ± 0.58 | 4.05 ± 0.94 |
| 90 min | 3.80 ± 0.32 | 3.71 ± 0.50 |
| 2 h | 3.76 ± 0.31 | 3.86 ± 0.65 |
| 3 h | 3.55 ± 0.33 | 3.43 ± 0.28 |
| 4 h | 2.88 ± 0.23 | 3.35 ± 0.22 |
| 5 h | 2.39 ± 0.23 | 2.85 ± 0.27 |
| 7 h | 2.15 ± 0.03 | 2.30 ± 0.26 |
| 12 h | 1.66 ± 0.22 | 1.76 ± 0.23 |
| 24 h | 0.86 ± 0.75 | 1.00 ± 0.18 |
| 30 h | 0.38 ± 0.09 | 0.68 ± 0.16 |

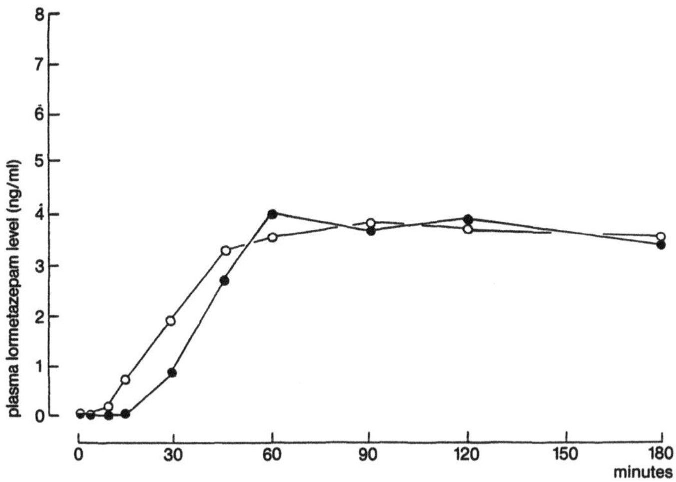


**Fig. 1.** Mean plasma lormetazepam concentration in groups of 8 male volunteers following sublingual (○) or oral (●) dosing with 1 mg lormetazepam

Following absorption, plasma lormetazepam was found to rapidly reach mean ($\pm$ s.d.) peak concentrations ($C_{p\,max}$ of $4.9 \pm 0.9$ ng/ml (range 3.7–6.6 ng/ml) and $5.2 \pm 1.7$ ng (range 3.6–7.4 ng/ml), for the sublingual and oral routes, respectively, there being no significant difference ($p > 0.05$) between these values. The time at which peak plasma lormetazepam concentrations occurred ($t_{max}$) ranged from 1–3 h (mean = $1.8 \pm 0.7$ h) following sublingual administration and 0.75–4 h (mean = $2.1 \pm 1.2$ h) after oral dosing. Once again, duspite a trend for $C_{p\,max}$ concentrations to be reached more rapidly after sublingual dosing, statistically, there was no difference ($p > 0.05$) between the $t_{max}$ values for the oral and sublingual groups.

Measurements of the area under each plasma concentration-time curve (0–30 h) was carried out using the trapezoid method, and found to be 47.98 and 52.88 h.ng/ml for sublingual and oral routes, respectively. Clearly the total amount of lormetazepam absorbed was similar for both dosage forms being independent of route of administration.

Following a fairly rapid decline in plasma lormetazepam concentrations, plasma levels then fell more slowly. The mean half-lives for elimination were calculated to be 13.0 and 13.8 h following sublingual and oral dosing, respectively.

## 4 Discussion

The results of this study clearly indicate that the plasma profiles of lormetazepam following sublingual and oral dosing are superimposable. While a trend towards a more rapid rate of absorption of lormetazepam was observed in seven of the eight volunteers receiving sublingual lormetazepam, this was not substantiated when the plasma level data was subjected to statistical analysis. Perhaps it should be stressed that volunteers who received lormetazepam orally, swallowed the tablet in a relatively fasted state. This favoured a speedy transit to the small intestine and consequently rapid absorption from this site. It can only be speculated upon at present that lormetazepam swallowed after an intake of food might exhibit delayed absorption and a subsequent delay in onset of hypnotic effect. In this instance, a delayed gastric emptying time might result in the plasma profile of lormetazepam being significantly different from that observed following sublingual dosing where the presence of food in the gastrointestinal tract is unimportant.

For drugs to be active sublingually, they must first cross the mucous membranes of the buccal cavity and subsequently pass into the blood stream. The process by which this occurs is generally by simple diffusion across a concentration gradient. Although the total area for absorption sublingually is comparatively small compared with the small intestine, where the absorption does take place, it does so rapidly. Since drug delivered via the mucous membranes enters the general circulation without first entering the portal system, the sublingual route is primarily used for drugs which are required to act rapidly and/or are either inactivated by the gastrointestinal tract when swallowed or undergo extensive first-pass metabolism (e.g. glyceryl trinitrate). In the case of lormetazepam, the drug is both stable in the gastrointestinal tract and does not undergo a substantial first-pass effect. This is confirmed by the fact that the plasma lormetazepam profiles following sublingual and oral dosing are virtually identical. Calculation of the area under each plasma concentration-versus-time curve clearly shows that the bioavailability of lormetazepam is independent of route of administration indicating that the drug is not metabolised to any great extent by the liver or gastrointestinal tract and consequently undergoes little first-pass effect, a fact previously reported by Hümpel et al. (1979). Since lormetazepam has been shown to be completely absorbed when swallowed orally (Hümpel et al. 1979), it may be assumed that the drug is also completely absorbed when administered sublingually.

The fact that identical values were obtained for the areas under each plasma concentration-versus-time curve was predictable. However, the shapes of the curves obtained after oral and sublingual dosing were not as expected. Firstly, one might have envisaged a more rapid appearance of lormetazepam in the plasma following sublingual dosing since the dosage form did not have to be firstly conveyed to its site of absorption (i.e. no lag phase prior to absorption). Secondly, peak plasma drug concentrations are usually higher after sublingual administration, although in the present study peak plasma levels were of the same order for the two routes of administration. Since elevated peak plasma concentrations are often associated with unwanted side-effects of the drug, the incidence of such induced side-effects is not likely to be increased on sublingual dosing.

It was also interesting to find that the excretion of lormetazepam was similar following oral and sublingual dosing. The mean elimination half-life values for the terminal phase of excretion were estimated to be 13.0 h and 13.8 h for the sublingual and oral groups, respectively. Clearly, lormetazepam is handled by the body in the same manner independent of the route of administration. This therefore allows one to predict a similar duration of drug effect whichever route of dosing is used clinically. It is perhaps reassuring that the half-life values determined in the present study are in good agreement with a mean value of 13.3 h reported on previously in a group of nine male volunteers who had received a single oral dose of 1 mg lormetazepam (Luscombe 1982). As is the case with orally administered lormetazepam, only minimal drug accumulation may be expected to occur with repeated sublingual dosing on a nightly basis, the elimination half-life being short enough to avoid such a phenomenon.

Perhaps the most important finding of this study is that lormetazepam is indeed absorbed sublingually, particularly when one considers that the dosage-form was identical to that swallowed orally. Not only is the plasma profile of lormetazepam independent of whether the tablet formulation is placed under the tongue or swallowed, the dosage form used (Noctamid® tablets) is tasteless, odourless, rapidly disintegrates (2–5 min) and is free from particulate residues, yet possesses all the characteristics of a tablet required to be swallowed orally. The advantage to a medical practitioner who is able to instruct a patient being unable to swallow tablets of any kind or size that he or she may take the same tablet sublingually, is immeasurable. The physician could be confident that whether the tablet be swallowed or used sublingually by the patient, the pharmacokinetic characteristics of lormetazepam would be the same thus ensuring a similar pharmacological profile. Furthermore, one can speculate that the induction period will remain similar even in a situation where the tablet is ultimately swallowed after an initial period of being dissolved under the tongue. Since problems of tablet swallowing are largely associated with geriatric patients, advantages of the sublingual/oral dosage form will be greatest amongst the elderly, who probably form the largest group of patients requiring a short-acting hypnotic. It is known that age-related changes in gastrointestinal function may modify absorption of orally administered drugs, although it must be emphasised that these effects have not yet been shown to have clinical significance. However, where they do take place and also where the patient is suffering from intestinal pathology which reduces drug absorption from the small intestine, then in these patients the alternative sublingual route of administration must surely prove particularly beneficial.

In conclusion, the findings in the present study indicate that following sublingual administration of a single dose of lormetazepam (Noctamid® 1 mg tablet), rapid absorption from the mucous membranes of the buccal cavity takes place. However, the speed with which lormetazepam appears in the plasma and the peak plasma levels attained are not statistically different from those observed in fasted volunteers receiving the same dose of lormetazepam swallowed orally. Likewise, plasma elimination of lormetazepam is similar in both instances. Indeed, the plasma concentration-versus-time curves following sublingual and oral dosing appeared to be superimposable indicating an identical pharmacokinetic profile of lormetazepam, independent of the route of administration.

## References

Dorow RG, Seidler J, Schneider HH (1982) A radioreceptor assay to study the affinity of benzodiazepines and their receptor binding activity in human plasma including their active metabolites. Br J Clin Pharmacol 13:561–565

Heidrich H, Ott H, Beach RC (1981) Lormetazepam – A benzodiazepine derivative without hangover effect? A double-blind study with chronic insomniacs in a general practice setting. Int J Clin Pharmacol Ther Toxicol 19:11–19

Hümpel M, Illi V, Milius W, Wendt H, Kurowski M (1979) The pharmacokinetics and biotransformation of the new benzodiazepine, lormetazepam, in humans. I. Absorption, distribution, elimination and metabolism of lormetazepam-5-$^{14}$C. Eur J Drug Metab Pharmacokinet 4:237–243

Jovanovic UV, Ott H, Heidrich H, Stephan K, Schratzer M (1980) Age-specific doses of lormetazepam as a night sedative in cases of chronic sleep disturbance. Waking and Sleeping 4:223–235

Luscombe DK (1982) Pharmacokinetics of lormetazepam. In: Benzodiazepines, sleep and daytime performance. Medicine Publishing Foundation, Oxford, pp 55–65

Oswald I, Adam K, Borrow S, Idzikowski C (1978) The effects of two hypnotics on sleep subjective feelings and skilled performance. Adv Biosci 9:199–202

# Pharmacokinetic and Clinical Studies with a Benzodiazepine Radioreceptor Assay

R. Dorow[1]

**Contents**



**Abstract**

Since the presence of benzodiazepine (BD) receptors was demonstrated in mammalian brain tissue, simple, sensitive and rapid techniques have been established to use BD-receptor preparations for specific radioreceptor assays (RRA). The RRA allows in vitro estimations of receptor affinity and concentration of BD in biological material, e.g. the time course of total BD binding activity in plasma (parent compound and active metabolites) may be evaluated.

Several studies in volunteers with short and long-acting BD used as sedatives and hypnotics including diazepam (DZP), flunitrazepam (FNZ), flurazepam (FZP), lormetazepam (LMZ), oxazepam, temazepam and triazolam indicate that pharmacokinetic data (e.g. elimination half-lives of receptor active compounds) concur with the results obtained from other methods, if active metabolites are taken into account. For the evaluation of BD long-term and hangover effects in two placebo controlled double-blind studies (placebo vs. 1 mg and 2 mg LMZ, 2 mg FNZ, 30 mg FZP, 10 mg DZP) BD-binding equivalents and pharmaco-EEG recordings, subjective state, psychomotor as well as cognitive function were determined by standardized methods up to 154 hours following drug administration. Compared to placebo a distinct long-lasting increase in the relative power in $\beta$-frequencies (12.5–30 Hz) and an impairment of psychomotor performance could be evidenced up to 12 h following FNZ and FZP intake. These effects correspond to the BD-binding activity in plasma.

These findings indicate that BD-receptor preparations as used for the RRA are valuable tools to investigate binding affinities and pharmacokinetic properties of BD. Plasma levels of RRA active material may reflect a better correspondence to some clinical effects of BD than levels of the parent compound alone.

**Key Words**

Benzodiazepines/Binding affinities/Pharmaco-EEG/Pharmacokinetics/Radioreceptor assay.

1 Research Laboratories, Schering AG, D-1000 Berlin 65, FRG

Psychopharmacology Supplementum 1
Editors: I. Hindmarch, H. Ott and T. Roth

# 1 Introduction

Specific binding sites with high affinity for benzodiazepines have been characterized in the mammalian brain (Squires and Braestrup 1977; Möhler and Okada 1977). These receptors are localized on synaptosomal membranes of nerve cells and are functionally linked to a GABA-receptor/chloride ionophore in a supramolecular complex (Tallman et al. 1980; see Fig. 1). Benzodiazepines and other chemically nonrelated compounds with benzodiazepine-like pharmacological profiles act via this complex by increasing chloride conductance. Recently it was shown that benzodiazepine receptor ligands with high specific affinity for the receptor may have an inverse active profile of the known benzodiazepines (inverse agonist), i.e. they elicit anxiety in humans (Dorow 1982; Dorow et al. 1983) and some even induce convulsions in animals (Braestrup et al. 1982).

There are also receptor antagonists available which lack pharmacological effects, but reverse both the effects of agonists and inverse agonists (Darragh et al. 1981; Hunkeler et al. 1981; Doenicke et al. 1982). Therefore, clinical effects of benzodiazepine receptor ligands are not only dependent on receptor affinity, but also on receptor efficacy. In general, pharmacokinetic parameters determine the duration of action of benzodiazepines.

When used as hypnotics, benzodiazepines may impair physical and mental performance the following day(s) in the form of hangover or rebound effects (Johnson and Chernic 1982; Morgan and Oswald 1982; Kales et al. 1983). In order to measure benzodiazepine plasma levels including their active metabolites and compare these and kinetic parameters with immediate and long-lasting

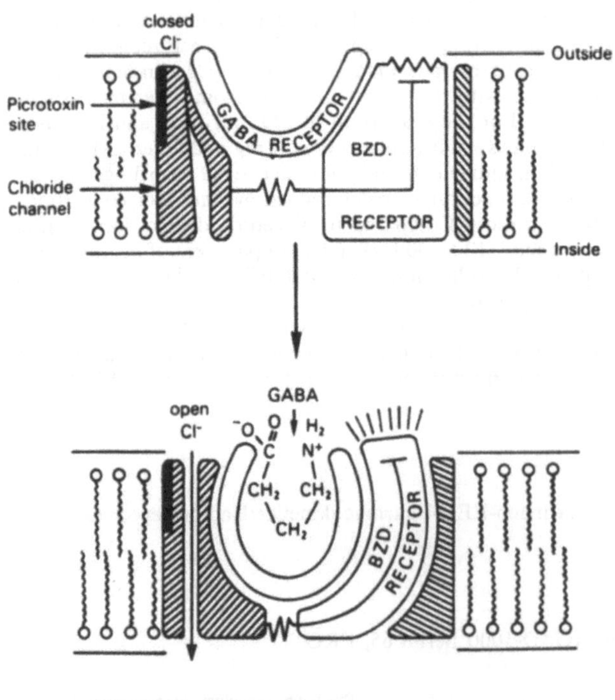


**Fig. 1.** Model of the GABA-benzodiazepine-chloride ionophore receptor complex. Occupation of GABA receptor induces an allosteric change in the conformation of benzodiazepine recognition site resulting in increased receptor affinity for benzodiazepines [adapted from Braestrup and Nielsen, 1980, ArzneimForsch/Drug Res 30 (I), Nr. 5a]

clinical effects a radioreceptor assay (RRA) for benzodiazepines was developed (Lund 1981; Dorow et al. 1982a).

## 2 The Benzodiazepine Radioreceptor Assay

Standard analytic methods for benzodiazepines like gas-chromatography coupled with electron-capture detection (GC-EC) (Greenblatt 1978) and HPLC (Brodie et al. 1978) are elaborate, time-consuming and require sophisticated technical equipment; they are therefore restricted to specialized laboratories. Radioimmunoassay (RIA) techniques are not generally available, as they depend on antibodies being formed for the benzodiazepine under investigation (Bourne et al. 1978; Hümpel et al. 1980). These methods allow the determination of only one compound at a time, which is important for kinetic investigations, but is not satisfactory when the correlation with clinical effects is investigated. The metabolism of benzodiazepines may produce a number of active metabolites which contribute to the clinical effects of the parent compound or form even the main active component, and may therefore determine the course of action.

Recent knowledge and understanding of receptors arose from technical advances and the development of specific radioligand receptor binding assays. Rapid filtration and centrifugation methods and ligands labelled with very high specific activity made it easy to investigate a number of membrane and cell preparations for receptors. These techniques generated new information on the biochemical characterization of binding sites. An approach to apply these methods in a different way was to develop quantitative assays for hormones, neurotransmitters or drugs.

Radioreceptor assays (RRA) have been used to determine, for example, ACTH (Lefkowitz et al. 1970), neuroleptic (Creese and Snyder 1977), opoid (Villiger et al. 1981), glucucorticoid (Lan and Baxter 1982) and steroid (Korenman 1970) binding activity in biological samples. Only few drug RRA have been developed and the method has not yet been fully exploited. RRA are comparable to RIA in that drug or other ligands can be determined by competition with a specific radioactive ligand ("tracer") for the recognition site. In contrast to the RIA, where the ligand is bound to an immunoglobulin, the RRA resembles a "bioassay" as the binding site is a specific receptor which may discriminate different ligands by affinity. The tracer is normally a high affinity prototype of the endogenous or exogenous compound. When samples containing unlabelled receptor binding substances are added to the incubation mixture, radioactive tracers will be displaced competitively from the binding sites as a function of both their concentration and receptor affinity (Fig. 2). Thus, for quantitative assays the amount of unknown receptor binding substance can be calculated by determining its inhibition of radioligand binding and comparing it to the inhibition produced by known quantities of unlabelled ligands. Benzodiazepines may be determined from body fluids and tissues including blood, urine and CSF.

Dry and stable (lyophilized) receptor preparations have become commercially available (Ferrosan, Denmark). They have binding characteristics that are similar to fresh brain membrane preparations (Lund 1981). Specimens are extracted

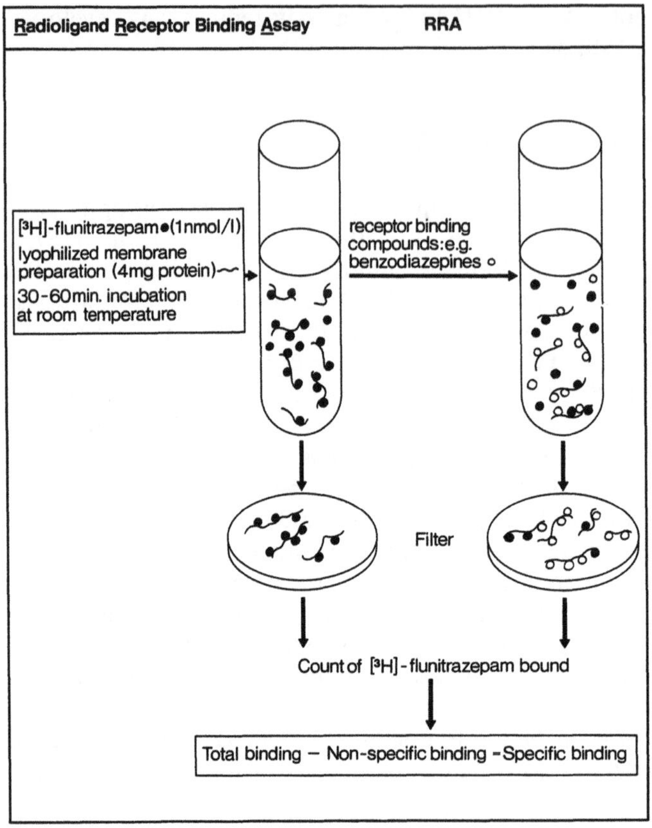


**Fig. 2.** Scheme of procedure for the benzodiazepine radioreceptor assay

and incubated at room temperature for 30–60 min with a mixture of $^3$H-flunitrazepam (1 nmol/1 = 50 nCi) and a benzodiazepine receptor suspension in a sodium phosphate buffer. The mixture is then passed through a glass-fibre filter and the radioactivity on the filter is determined by liquid scintillation counting (for details see Lund 1981; Dorow et al. 1982a). Good correlations between results by specific methods like e.g. GC-EC and the RRA have been demonstrated (Lund 1981; Skolnick et al. 1979; Jochemsen et al. 1982). The RRA method displays an accuracy comparable to that of GC-EC techniques. Sensitivity of the RRA is usually defined as the amount of substance that will displace at least 20% of the radioligand. Below this limit variability in displacement is considerably increased. The RRA is feasible for most clinical or forensic laboratories from a methodological point of view. The technique is not time-consuming and does not require sophisticated equipment. Moreover, the use of tracers with high specific affinity and activity, e.g. $^3$H-flunitrazepam allows assay performance at room temperature. The lyophilized tracer and the dry receptor preparation eliminate the need for fresh or frozen brain tissue, which adds to the simplicity and speed of the method. In addition, the method is sensitive to plasma concentrations of benzodiazepines with a high clinical potency, i.e. to a low therapeutic dose, as the sensitivity of the RRA is enhanced in proportion to the receptor affinity of these compounds.

## 3 Applications of the Benzodiazepine RRA

### 3.1 The RRA as Research Tool for New Drugs

Once a bioassay is available, new substances can be screened in search of some specific activity in this system. In fact, in modern drug research binding assays are in first place when new drugs are screened. This in part is due to the simple technique generally involved in performing the assays. After benzodiazepine receptors had become available for binding techniques a number of drugs binding to these receptors, but unrelated to benzodiazepines in their chemical structures, were detected. A limitation, however, to binding studies in general is that no indication is given as to whether a drug is functionally active at the specific binding site and, if this applies, whether it acts as an agonist or an antagonist. One of the most interesting findings was the isolation of β-carboline-3-carboxylic-acid-ethyl ester (β-CCE) from human urine. At the time of its discovery β-CCE was thought to be an endogenous ligand for the benzodiazepine receptor (Nielsen et al. 1979). It turned out to be an isolation artefact originating from the extraction of the receptor-inactive β-carboline carboxylic acid in ethanol. However, β-CCE was found to be a potent ligand to the benzodiazepine receptor with a pharmacological profile different from the known benzodiazepines in that it not only antagonizes the effects of benzodiazepines, but has a pharmacological activity of its own (Tenen and Hirsch 1980). As its metabolic breakdown is rather rapid, i.e. its half-life is short, a number of more stable compounds were synthesized, one of which β-carboline-3-carboxylic-acid-monomethyl-amide (FG 7142) with a similar pharmacological profile was investigated in animals (Petersen et al. 1982) and humans (Dorow et al. 1983). Meanwhile a number of β-carbolines have been found to be agonists, receptor antagonists and inverse agonists at the benzodiazepine receptor (Braestrup et al. 1982; Dorow et al. 1983; Hunkeler et al. 1981; Jensen et al. 1983).

### 3.2 Estimation of Binding Affinities

Radioligand receptor binding studies may be used to evaluate binding affinities of receptor ligands. These affinities are expressed as concentrations at which 50% of the tracer is displaced ($IC_{50}$) or as inhibitor constants ($K_i$). Receptor affinities can be correlated to pharmacological and clinical effects in animals and humans (Möhler and Okada 1977; Braestrup and Squires 1978; Malick and Enna 1979). Fig. 3 shows the correlation between the recommended clinical dose and the receptor affinity as expressed by the $K_i$ of various benzodiazepines (Dorow et al. 1982a). Medazepam which does not accommodate to this correlation is a prodrug with very low benzodiazepine receptor affinity. It is metabolized to the active drugs diazepam and desmethyldiazepam and, therefore, is effective in doses similar to those which are known to be the therapeutic ones for desmethyl-

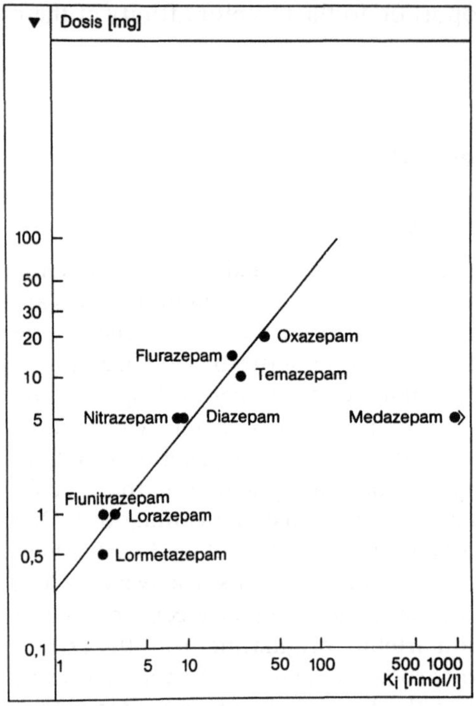


**Fig. 3.** Correlation of the lowest recommended clinical dose of benzodiazepines with their in vitro receptor affinities ($K_i$) (from Dorow et al. 1982a)

diazepam (Rieder and Rentsch 1968). The in vitro/in vivo correlations of this nature may even be helpful for drug trials in humans in order to establish approximate doses of new benzodiazepines or benzodiazepine-like agents.

## 3.3 Determination of Plasma Levels of Benzodiazepine Receptor Ligands

Standard analytical methods for benzodiazepines allow measurements of only one compound at a time, which is essential for kinetic investigations of the parent drug, but is not satisfactory when the correlation to clinical effects is being assessed. Metabolism may produce a number of active metabolites which contribute to the clinical effects of the parent compound or are even the main active components as is known from the examples of diazepam and flurazepam. These active metabolites may determine the time course of clinical effects. The RRA is a suitable method to measure the concentration of all receptor binding substances, i.e. parent compound(s) and/or active metabolite(s) in body fluids and tissue.

We have studied the time course of benzodiazepine receptor ligand concentrations following the oral administration of a number of benzodiazepines. The results of two studies in which lormetazepam (1 mg), flunitrazepam (2 mg), diazepam (10 mg) (study I) and 1 mg lormetazepam, 50 mg oxazepam, 20 or 30 mg temazepam and 0.5 mg triazolam were given orally are shown in Figs. 4 and 5 (Dorow et al. 1982a; Dorow and Lund 1983). Blood was drawn from an indwelling catheter up to 154 h (study I) or 48 h (study II) post application.

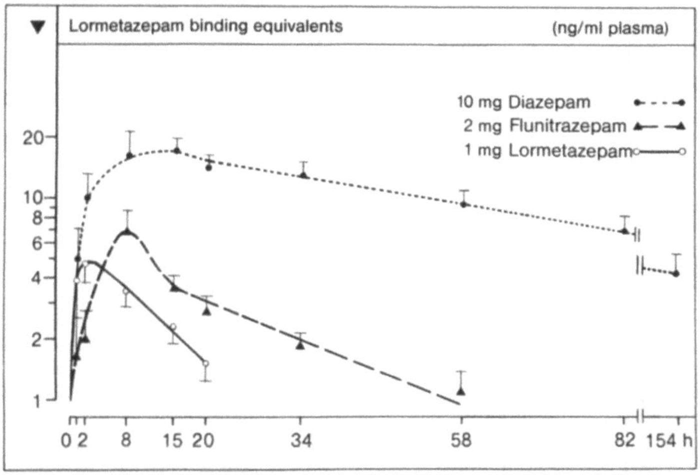


**Fig. 4.** Time course of plasma benzodiazepine binding equivalents after single oral dose of 1 mg lormetazepam, 2 mg flunitrazepam or 10 mg diazepam expressed as ng lormetazepam/ml plasma. Mean of eight volunteers; bars indicate s.e. mean (from Dorow et al. 1982a)

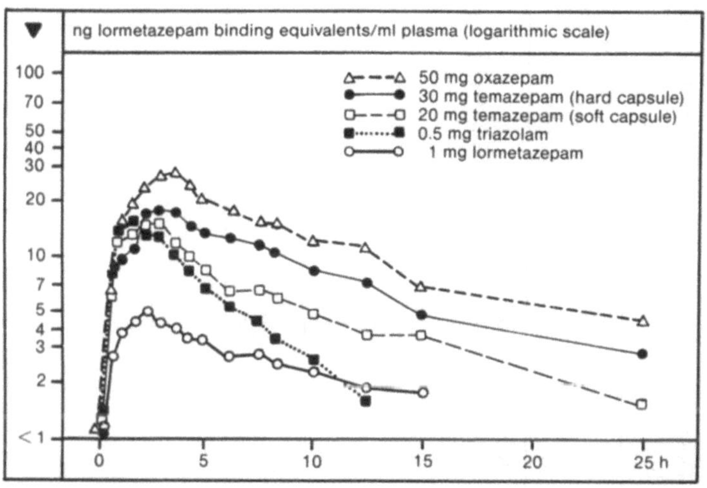


**Fig. 5.** Time course of benzodiazepine (ng lormetazepam/ml plasma) binding equivalents in plasma after single oral doses of lormetazepam 1 mg, oxazepam 50 mg, temazepam 20 mg (soft capsule), temazepam 30 mg (hard capsule), and triazolam 0.5 mg. Mean of 10 volunteers

A clear advantage of the RRA is obvious in that all benzodiazepines can be referred to the same standard curve yielding comparable measures expressed as receptor binding equivalents. These composite measures of both affinity and concentration form a correlative parameter with clinical effects which is more valid than the concentration of the parent drug alone. The elimination half-lives as determined by the RRA and evaluated by a regression analysis of the semi-logarithmic graph and the receptor affinities ($K_i$) are presented in Table 1.

**Table 1.** Elimination half-lives and receptor affinities ($K_i$) of benzodiazepines and their major active metabolites

| Benzodiazepines<br>Major active metabolites | Dose [mg] | $K_i$ [nmol/l] | Elimination half-life [h][a] | | References |
|---|---|---|---|---|---|
| | | | RRA | Other methods | |
| Lormetazepam | 1–2 | 2.4 | 9.1 (6.7–16.9) | 10 (7–14) | Hümpel et al. 1980 |
| Temazepam | 20 | 24 | 8.2 (4.5–11.4) | 8.4 | Fuccella et al. 1977 |
| Oxazepam | 50 | 37 | 8.2 (3.6–11.7) | 8.2 (5.9–12.9) | Alván et al. 1977 |
| Triazolam | 0.5 | 0.5 | | 2.3 (1.7–3.0) | Eberts et al. 1981 |
| 1-Hydroxymethyltriazolam | – | – | 3.8 (2.4–4.7) | – | |
| 4-Hydroxytriazolam | – | – | | – | |
| Flunitrazepam | 2 | 2.4 | | 14 (9–25) | Boxenbaum et al. 1978 |
| 7-amino derivate | – | – | 23 (15–52) | 23 | Wendt 1976 |
| N-Desmethyl derivate | – | 7.3 | | 31 | Wendt 1976 |
| Flurazepam | 30 | 22 | 71 (29–116) | (1.6–5.3) | Anderjan et al. 1980 |
| Desalkylflurazepam | – | – | | (47–100) | Kaplan and de Silva 1973 |
| Diazepam | 10 | 9.3 | 63 (34–180) | 32 (41–46) | Kaplan et al. 1973 |
| N-Desmethyldiazepam | – | 13 | | (59–99) | Kaplan et al. 1973 |

[a] Mean and range

Interestingly, all 3-hydroxylated benzodiazepines (lormetazepam, temazepam and oxazepam) which are readily glucuronidized (phase II reactions) in the 3-position have similar elimination half-lives of 8–10 h in healthy young subjects. The times to peak concentrations ($t_{max}$) differ slightly. In the mean triazolam concentrations peak after 60 min (range 30–120 min), lormetazepam after 90 min (range 30 – 300 min), temazepam (soft gelatine capsule) after 120 min (range 45–240 min), temazepam (hard gelatine capsule) after 120 min (range 45–420 min) and oxazepam after 120 min (range 45–300 min). The data for temazepam are at variance with $t_{max}$ values reported in a study by Fuccella et al. (1977) in which the Scherer soft gelatine capsule containing temazepam in a solution of propyleneglycol had a considerably shorter time to peak value ($t_{max}$ = 50 min) than temazepam in hard gelatine capsules ($t_{max}$ = 86 min). Triazolam has a considerably shorter half-life ($t_{1/2}$ = 3.8 h) than the 3-hydroxylated compounds which is in agreement with published data (Eberts et al. 1981). Although active metabolites (1-methylhydroxy- and 4-hydroxy-triazolam) are formed, they do not contribute to the half-life of benzodiazepine binding equivalents to a major extent (Table 1). Jochemsen et al. (1982) found a good correlation between RRA values and triazolam concentrations evaluated by GC-EC. This finding supports our own results with respect to the absence of major active long-lasting metabolites. However, benzodiazepines which form longer-lasting metabolites as, for instance, diazepam, flurazepam and flunitrazepam, have a terminal half-life and clearance rate of benzodiazepine receptor binding equivalents which differ markedly from those of the parent compound. The terminal half-life of RRA assayable material is considerably longer than that of the parent compound.

## 4 Correlation of Pharmacokinetic Data as Determined by the RRA to Clinical Effects

Quantitative relationships between biological effects and drug plasma concentrations are difficult to establish as concentrations of benzodiazepines, including the active metabolites, have to be considered. Plasma levels do not necessarily reflect the conditions at the CNS receptor site. In part, this situation will be improved by investigating benzodiazepine-binding equivalent plasma levels (Horowski and Dorow 1982). Factors influencing pharmacokinetics of benzodiazepines, like protein binding, volume of distribution, clearance, disease and age as well as single dose vs. chronic treatment have to be considered when correlations between kinetics and pharmacodynamics are to be established.

Depending on the concentration and receptor affinity, the plasma concentration time curve, as evaluated by the RRA, and the clinical effect are determined by the active metabolite. Desmethyldiazepam, e.g., has 70% receptor affinity of diazepam and is found in large concentrations after diazepam treatment (Kaplan et al. 1973), which may add considerably to the clinical effect. This also holds true for flurazepam, the major active metabolite of which, desalkylflurazepam (Kaplan and de Silva 1973), is well known to account for the clinical profile of the drug. Various authors tried to correlate clinical effects of benzodiazepines with plasma levels, measuring the parent compound only. Results from these studies, however, are contradictory. Following diazepam and desmethyldiazepam administration, a correlation of plasma levels with the anxiolytic action and side effects was reported (Dasberg et al. 1974; Curry 1974), whereas other authors (Bond et al. 1977) were unable to see any clear relationship in these parameters. For flunitrazepam, which also produces active metabolites, a significant correlation of plasma drug levels and impairment of fine motor coordination, memory performance and power of concentration was reported (Amrein 1978), whereas Wickstrøm et al. (1980) were unable to find a correlation between clinical effects and plasma levels. In some studies with compounds lacking active metabolites, satisfactory correlations were observed (Kurowski et al. 1982). Also, when specific aspects of brain function, e.g. velocity of saccadic eye movements or EEG effects were analysed, a relationship to benzodiazepine plasma levels was found (Bittencourt et al. 1981; Fink et al. 1976).

As an index for CNS activity of benzodiazepines, EEG measurements may be of value because functional changes in different frequency bands, especially in the relative $\beta$-power, concur with benzodiazepine plasma levels. In order to establish the relationship of clinical and hangover effects of benzodiazepines, a number of studies in healthy volunteers were performed in our laboratories, which included pharmaco-EEG, psychomotor tests and visual analogue scales as investigational tools (Ott 1984). Especially for lormetazepam, flunitrazepam and flurazepam a sound correlation of terminal half-lives and benzodiazepine activities in plasma with an increase of $\beta$-frequencies (12.5–30 Hz) in the power spectra of the pharmaco-EEG (Dorow et al. 1982b; N. Sauerbrey, thesis; Figs. 6 and 7) could be established. Long-lasting enhancement of fast frequencies ($\beta$ = 12.5–30 Hz) seen up to 60 hours following treatment with 30 mg flurazepam, but not after 2 mg

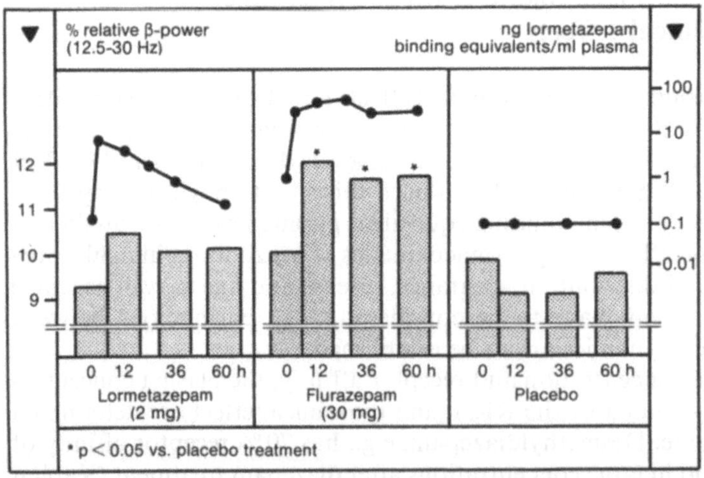


**Fig. 6.** Mean relative power of the beta-frequency band (12.5–30 Hz) from EEG and mean benzodiazepine plasma levels (lormetazepam binding equivalents/ml plasma) in 15 healthy volunteers at various times after single oral administration of lormetazepam 2 mg, flurazepam 30 mg and placebo. Significant levels (* = $p < 0.05$ vs. placebo treatment) were evaluated after analysis of variance followed by Tukey test (results by N. Sauerbrey, thesis)

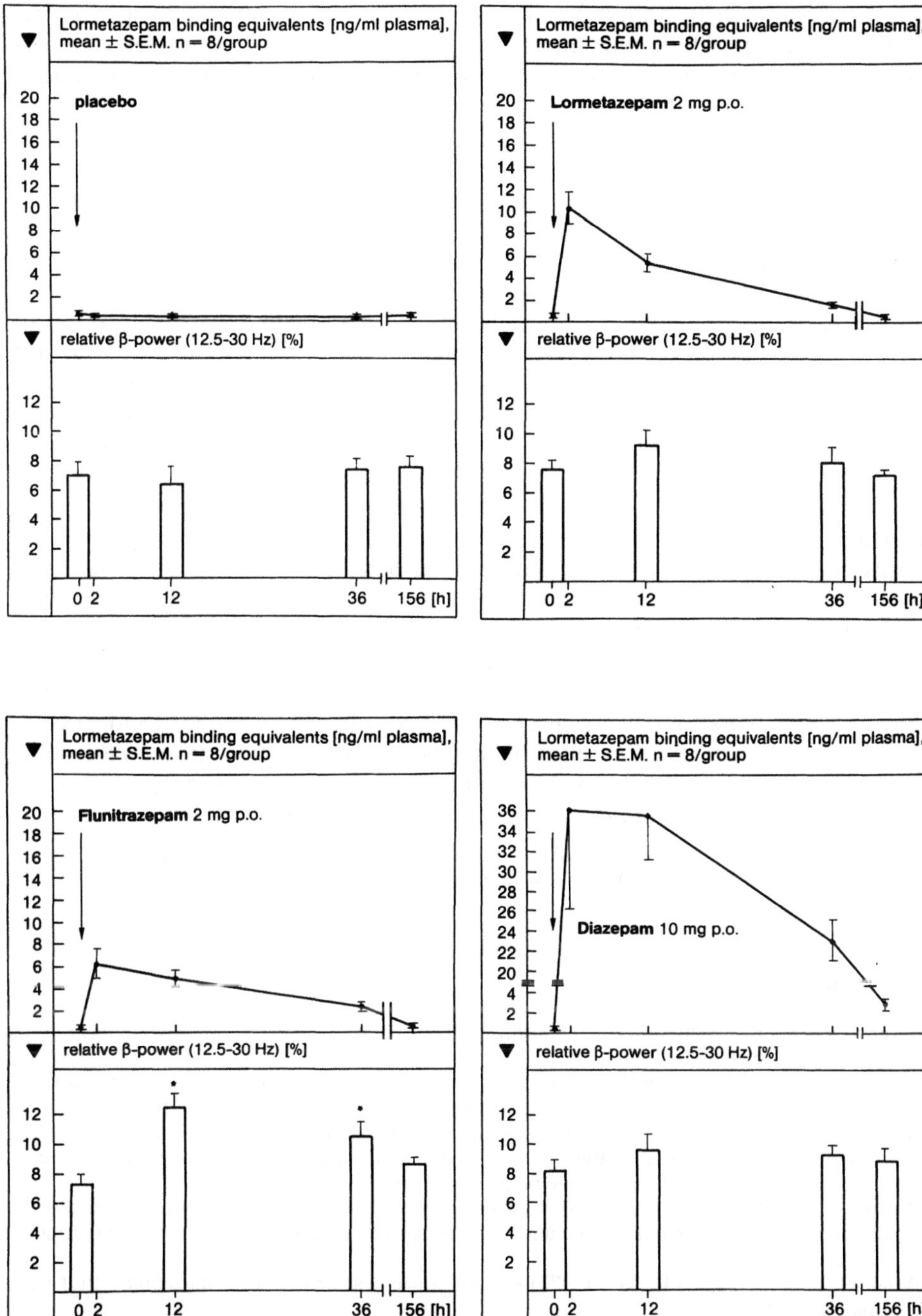


**Fig. 7.** Benzodiazepine plasma levels (mean ± SEM) expressed as ng lormetazepam binding equivalents/ml plasma after single oral doses of 2 mg lormetazepam, 2 mg flunitrazepam, 10 mg diazepam or placebo, and the relative power of the $\beta$-band (12.5–30 Hz) from the EEG

lormetazepam (Fig. 6), correlate with high levels of receptor binding material after flurazepam. The augmentation of low voltage fast frequencies is short-lasting after lormetazepam, but is protracted (diazepam) and more pronounced after flunitrazepam and flurazepam. Also sleep latency and sleep quality have corresponded to the time course of benzodiazepine binding equivalents in plasma (Dorow et al. 1982b; Ott 1984). After diazepam treatment, however, long-lasting high plasma levels of benzodiazepine binding equivalents did not account for measurable hangover effects 36 h p.a. (Fig. 7). Benzodiazepine binding equivalents in plasma need not reflect brain levels at the receptor site. Other factors, for example the development of tolerance or different pharmacological, e.g. antagonistic effects of the active metabolite desmethyldiazepam (Elsass et al. 1980), may be involved. However, benzodiazepine binding equivalents do not necessarily reflect the pharmacological efficacy of the compounds, but only concentration and affinity to the benzodiazepine receptor. For example, administration of the benzodiazepine antagonist Ro 15-1788 with high affinity to the benzodiazepine receptor leads to significant RRA-measurable plasma levels, although no clinical effects of the compound itself were reported (Hunkeler et al. 1981; Darragh et al. 1981). A lacking correlation between clinical effects and plasma levels may also become evident with partial benzodiazepine receptor agonists.

The RRA may also be used routinely for the control of the patient's compliance to drug intake in the course of clinical trials or, e.g., in the case of clonazepam for monitoring therapeutic levels in epileptic patients. Moreover, the RRA has been used successfully in forensic medicine to determine benzodiazepines in the blood of drivers checked for alcohol consumption (Steentoft et al. 1981). In addition, the occurence of benzodiazepines in intoxicated patients is readily assessed by this method. Also, in psychiatric patients and drug addicts, the RRA is well-suited for the discovery of benzodiazepine abuse.

*Acknowledgements.* The author wishes to thank A. Hammel, R. Herrmann, U. Hippler, C. Knittel for their excellent technical assistance, and E. Staab-Renner for her patience and help in preparing the manuscript.

## References

Alván G, Siwers B, Vessman J (1977) Pharmacokinetics of oxazepam in healthy volunteers. Acta Pharmacol Toxicol (Kbh) 40:40

Anderjan R, Fritz P, Mattern R (1980) Zur Bedeutung des Nachweises und der Pharmakokinetik von Flurazepam-Metaboliten in menschlichem Blut. ArzneimForsch/Drug Res 30:1944

Amrein R (1978) Zur Pharmakokinetik und zum Metabolismus von Flunitrazepam. In: Ahnefeld FW, Bergmann H, Burri C et al. (eds) Anaesthesiology and intensive care medicine, vol 17. Springer, Berlin Heidelberg New York, pp 9–24

Bittencourt PRM, Wade P, Smith AT, Richens A (1981) The relationship between peak velocity of saccadic eye movement and serum benzodiazepine concentration. Br J Clin Pharmacol 12:523

Bond AJ, Hailey DM, Lader MH (1977) Plasma concentrations of benzodiazepines. Br J Clin Pharmacol 4:51

Bourne RC, Robinson JD, Teale JD (1978) A simple radioimmunoassay for plasma diazepam and its application to single dose studies in man. Br J Pharmacol 63:371

Boxenbaum HG, Posmanter HN, Macasieb T, et al. (1978) Pharmacokinetics of flunitrazepam following single and multiple-dose administration to healthy human subjects. J Pharmacokinetic Biopharm 6:283–293

Braestrup C, Squires RF (1978) Pharmacological characterization of benzodiazepine receptors in the brain. Eur J Pharmacol 48:263

Braestrup C, Schmiechen R, Neef G, Nielsen M, Petersen EN (1982) Interaction of convulsive ligands with benzodiazepine receptors. Science 216:1241–1243

Brodie RR, Chasseaud LF, Taylor T (1978) High-performance liquid chromatographic determination of benzodiazepines in human plasma. J Chromatogr 150:361

Creese J, Snyder SH (1977) A simple and sensitive radioreceptor assay for antischizophrenic drugs in blood. Nature 270:180

Curry SH (1974) Concentration-effect relationships with major and minor tranquillizers. Clin Pharmacol Ther 16:192

Darragh A, Lambe R, Scully M, Brick I, O'Boyle C, Downie WW (1981) Investigation in man of the efficacy of a benzodiazepine antagonist, Ro 15-1788. Lancet 2:8–10

Dasberg HH, von der Kleijn E, Guelen PJR, van Praag HM (1974) Plasma concentrations of diazepam and of its metabolite N-desmethyldiazepam in relation to anxiolytic effect. Clin Pharmacol Ther 15:473

Doenicke A, Suttmann H, Kugler J, Kapp W, Wolf R (1982) Pilot study of a benzodiazepine antagonist. Br J Anaesth 54:1132

Dorow R (1982) β-Carboline monomethylamide causes anxiety in man. Abstracts, vol 1:175, Collegium Internationale Neuro-Psychopharmacologicum, 13th CINP Congress, Jerusalem

Dorow RG, Seidler J, Schneider HH (1982a) A radioreceptor assay to study the affinity of benzodiazepines and their receptor binding activity in human plasma including their active metabolites. Br J Clin Pharmacol 13:561

Dorow R, Hammer K, Ott H, Sauerbrey N (1982b) Correlation of benzodiazepine plasma levels with hangover effects as evaluated by radioreceptor assay, EEG and psychomotor performance. Abstracts, Sixth Eur Congr Sleep Research, Zurich, p 99

Dorow R, Horowski R, Paschelke G, Amin M, Braestrup C (1983) Severe anxiety induced by FG 7142, a β-carboline ligand for benzodiazepine receptors. Lancet 8341:98–99

Dorow R, Lund J (1983) The benzodiazepine radioreceptor assay – its use for pharmacokinetic and clinical studies. In: Benzodiazepines, sleep and daytime performance. (Medicine Publishing Foundation Symposium Series). Medicine Publishing Foundation, Oxford, pp 67–76

Eberts FS, Philopoulos Y, Reineke LM, Vliek RW (1981) Triazolam disposition. Clin Pharmacol Ther 29:81

Elsass P, Hendel J, Hvidberg EF, Hansen T, Gymoese E, Rathje J (1980) Kinetics and neuropsychologic effects of IV diazepam in the presence and absence of its active N-desmethyl metabolite in humans. Psychopharmacology (Berlin) 70:307

Fink M, Irwin P, Weinfeld RE, Schwartz MA, Conney AH (1976) Blood levels and electroencephalographic effects of diazepam and bromazepam. Clin Pharmacol Ther 20:184

Fuccella M, Bolcioni G, Tamassia V, Ferrario L, Tognoni G (1977) Human pharmacokinetics and bioavailability of temazepam administered in soft gelatin capsules. Eur J Clin Pharmacol 12:383

Greenblatt DJ (1978) Simultaneous gas-chromatographic analysis for diazepam and its major metabolite, desmethyldiazepam, with use of double internal standardization. Clin Chem 24:1838

Horowski R, Dorow R (1982) Die Bedeutung pharmakokinetischer Befunde für die klinische Wirkung von Benzodiazepinen. Internist 23:632

Hümpel M, Nieuweboer B, Milius W, Hanke H, Wendt H (1980) The pharmacokinetics of lormetazepam. II. Radioimmunological determinations in plasma and urine of young and elderly volunteers: First-pass effect. Clin Pharmacol Ther 28:673

Hunkeler W, Möhler H, Pieri L, Polc P, Bonetti EP, Cumin R, Schaffner R, Haefely W (1981) Selective antagonists of benzodiazepines. Nature 290:514

Jensen LH, Petersen EN, Braestrup C (1983) Audiogenic seizures in DBA/2 mice discriminate sensitively between low efficacy benzodiazepine receptor agonists and inverse agonists. Life Sci 33:393–399

Jochemsen R, Horbach GJMJ, Breimer DD (1982) Assay of nitrazepam and triazolam in plasma by a radioreceptor technique and comparison with a gaschromatographic method. Res Commun Chem Pathol Pharmacol 35:259

Johnson LC, Chernic DA (1982) Sedative-hypnotics and human performance. Psychopharmacology (Berlin) 76:101–113

Kales A, Soldatos CR, Bixler EO, Kales JD (1983) Rebound insomnia and rebound anxiety: A review. Pharmacology (Berlin) 26:121–137

Kaplan SA, de Silva JAF (1973) Blood level profile in man following chronic administration of flurazepam hydrochloride. J Pharm Sci 62:1932

Kaplan SA, Jack ML, Alexander K, Weinfeld RE (1973) Pharmacokinetic profile of diazepam in man following single intravenous and oral and chronic oral administrations. J Pharm Sci 62:1789

Korenman SG (1970) Relation between estrogen inhibitory activity and binding to cytosol of rabbit and human uterus. Endocrinology 87:1119

Kurowski M, Ott H, Herrmann WM (1982) Relationship between EEG dynamics and pharmacokinetics of the benzodiazepine lormetazepam. Pharmacopsychiat 15:77

Lan NC, Baxter JD (1982) A radioreceptor assay for direct measurement of plasma free glucucorticoid activity. J Clin Endocrinol Metab 55:516

Lefkowitz R, Roth J, Pastan I (1970) Radioreceptor assay of adrenocorticotropic hormone: New approach to assay of polypeptide hormones in plasma. Science 170:633

Lund J (1981) Radioreceptor assay for benzodiazepines in biological fluids using a new dry and stable receptor preparation. Scand J Clin Lab Invest 41:275

Malick JB, Enna SJ (1979) Comparative effects of benzodiazepines and non-benzodiazepine anxiolytics on biochemical and behavioral tests predictive of anxiolytic activity. Commun Psychopharmacol 3:245

Morgan K, Oswald I (1982) Anxiety caused by a short-life hypnotic. Br Med J 284:942

Möhler H, Okada T (1977) Benzodiazepine receptor: demonstration in the central nervous system. Science 198:849–851

Nielsen M, Gredal O, Braestrup C (1979) Some properties of $^3$H-diazepam displacing activity from human urine. Life Sci 25:679–686

Ott H (1984) Are electroencephalographic and psychomotor measures sensitive in detecting residual sequelae of benzodiazepine hypnotics. In: Hindmarch I, Ott H, Roth T (eds) Sleep, benzodiazepines and performance: Experimental methodologies and research prospects. See this volume, pp 133–151

Petersen EN, Paschelke G, Kehr W, Nielsen M, Braestrup C (1982) Does the reversal of the anticonflict effect of phenobarbital by β-CCE and FG 7142 indicate benzodiazepine receptor-mediated anxiogenic properties? Eur J Pharmacol 82:217–221

Rieder J, Rentsch G (1968) Metabolismus und Pharmakokinetik des neuen Psychopharmakons 7-Chlor-2,3-dihydro-1-methyl-5-phenyl-1H-1,4-benzodiazepin (Ro 5-4556) beim Menschen. Drug Res 18:1545

Skolnick P, Goodwin FK, Paul SM (1979) A rapid and sensitive radioreceptor assay for benzodiazepine in plasma. Arch Gen Psychiatry 36:78

Squires RF, Braestrup C (1977) Benzodiazepine receptors in rat brain. Nature 266:732

Steentoft A, Worm K, Christensen H (1981) The frequency of benzodiazepines in blood samples received for blood alcohol determination in the Danish population for the period June 1978–June 1979. J Forensic Sci Soc 21:142

Tallman JF, Paul SM, Skolnick P, Gallager DW (1980) Receptors for the age of anxiety: pharmacology of the benzodiazepines. Science 207:274–281

Tenen SS, Hirsch JD (1980) β-Carboline-3-carboxylic acid ethyl ester antagonizes diazepam activity. Nature 288:609

Villiger JW, Boas RA, Taylor KM (1981) A radioreceptor assay for opiate drugs in human cerebrospinal fluid and plasma. Life Sci 29:229–233

Wendt G (1976) Schicksal des Hypnotikums Flunitrazepam im menschlichen Organismus. In: Huegin W, Hossli G, Gemperle M (eds) Bisherige Erfahrungen mit ‚Rohypnol' (Flunitrazepam) in der Anaesthesiologie und Intensiv-therapie. Editions Roche, Basel, p 27 ff

Wickstrøm E, Amrein R, Haefelfinger P, Hartmann D (1980) Pharmacokinetic and clinical observations on prolonged administration of flunitrazepam. Eur J Clin Pharmacol 17:189

# Modern Trends in the Investigation of New Hypnotics in Anaesthesia

A. Doenicke [1]

## Contents



## Abstract

Over the last 20 years standardized techniques have been employed for the investigation of intravenous hypnotics, psychotropic and neuroleptic drugs. Sleep has been studied with the help of EEG measures and side-effects have been evaluated by psychometric tests. The EEG is a proven parameter with regard to dosage determination and as objective means to find sleep-inducing quantities of drugs. By means of vigilosomnograms we have established dose-effect curves and have made comparisons between related drugs in the form of equivalence studies. From an anaesthesiological point of view controllability of a substance is determined by duration of effect (short- or long-acting) and by depth of sleep (light or deep states) achieved. By these criteria midazolam displays good controllability with regard to duration, but not in terms of depth of sleep, since it follows the "all-or-nothing" rule, even with 0.1 mg/kg following both intravenous or intramuscular injection. Lormetazepam, on the other hand, shows good controllability of depth of sleep from tranquillity via sedation to hypnosis, but duration of effect is less well controllable in that patients remain lightly asleep even after 2 h. According to the vigilosomnograms the lormetazepam/oxygen/nitrous oxide combination produced a super-added increase in the depth of the hypnotic effect. After droperidol the specific nitrous oxide component of the depth of sleep at $B_0$ stage was not exceeded. The development of benzodiazepine antagonists, which immediately counteract the benzodiazepine induced sleep and respiratory obstruction is a milestone in the area of CNS research.

## Key Words

Alpha blockade/Apnoea/Benzodiazepines/Benzodiazepine antagonists/Butyrophenones/Capnography/Circulation/Controllability/Diazepam/Droperidol/ECG/EEG/Flunitrazepam/Heart/Imidazodiazepine/Immunosuppression/Liberation of histamine/Lorazepam/Lormetazepam/Lormetazepam-oxygen-nitrous-oxide combination/Mental changes/Midazolam/Nightmares/Nitrous Oxide/Pancuronium/Propanidid/Psychometric tests/Vigilosomnogram.

---

1 Department of Anaesthesiology, University of Munich, D-8000 Munich, FRG

Psychopharmacology Supplementum 1
Editors: I. Hindmarch, H. Ott and T. Roth

## 1 Introduction

Different drugs have their own characteristic EEG pattern permitting classification of new substances. One must, however, qualify this by stating that the EEG primarily quantifies the depth of sleep, and that this is only conditionally applicable to the depth of anaesthesia. In addition to the depth of sleep, a record must also be made of the effect of a drug on the purely central control of circulation and respiration, and on direct and indirect peripheral effects. Pharmacological substances are closely controlled and monitored during testing to record all possible side-effects (for example, heart and circulation, liberation of histamine, immunosuppression, alpha blockade, irritation of the venous system, nightmares, mental changes, disturbed relationship to the environment).

As benzodiazepines add anxiety relieving, sedative and hypnotic components to their range of action, any investigative procedure is useful that allows one to differentiate and characterize individual members of their group.

The EEG has proved itself particularly useful in this respect as comparisons and judgements can be based on it. To start with, some investigations with regard to lorazepam may be mentioned (Doenicke et al. 1981). 1, 2, 3 and 4 mg/kg body weight of lorazepam were injected at a constant speed into each of three subjects resulting in characteristic pharmacodynamic behaviour (Fig. 1). Average induc-

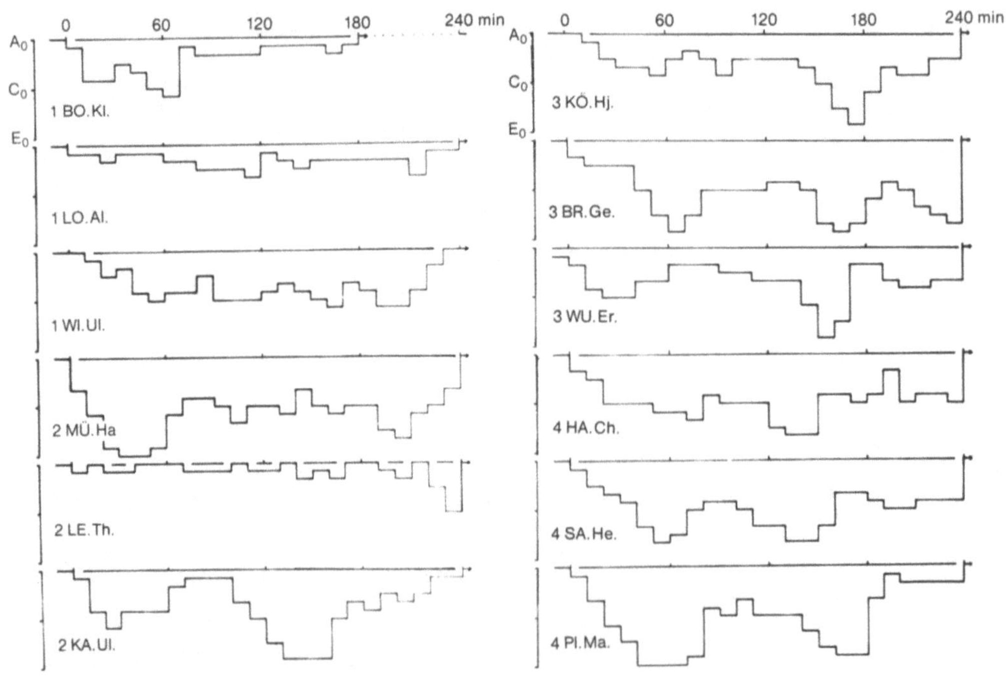


**Fig. 1.** Vigilosomnogram depicted in decades after four different dosages of lorazepam (1, 2, 3, 4 mg/70 kg body weight; three subjects for each dose group). The first period of deep sleep commenced after 60 min, and the second after 180 min. $A_0 - E_0$: different vigilosomnogram stages

tion time of sleep decreased with elevated dosage and the average duration of sleep increased. The standard deviation was lowest with 4 mg dosages.

## 2 Comparative Studies

In the course of further investigations based on the lorazepam profile, comparative studies were set up between 2 mg lorazepam, 7 mg diazepam and 1 mg lormetazepam per 70 kg body weight with regard to depth of sleep, latent period, individual scatter and duration of sleep, all evaluated statistically (Doenicke et al. 1981). With regard to sleep parameters, lormetazepam showed on the average vigilosomnogram (VSG) an onset of effect as rapid as that of diazepam (Fig. 2), but it produced appreciably deeper sleep which was maximal in the 40th minute with a slow fall-off in the 43rd minute. Judged by the average length of sleep (Fig. 3), lormetazepam was shown to be the most effective hypnotic.

Lorazepam proved to have a significantly longer time of sleep induction in the 1st to 12th minute ($p < 0.05$) compared with the other two substances, and a longer sleep effect, lasting from the 63rd to the 122nd minute ($p < 0.05$).

On an average the deepest sleep ($C_0$) was reached after 20 min with diazepam and lormetazepam, but only after 50 min with lorazepam (Fig. 4). Lormetazepam has advantages over lorazepam 2 mg and diazepam 7 mg in terms of onset of sleep, less individual differences, overall hypnotic effect and maximal depth of sleep.

In a further study, the hypnotic effect of the new benzodiazepine midazolam was established objectively (Doenicke et al. 1980). Midazolam differs from these substances not only by its water-solubility and kinetics, but also by its pharmaco-

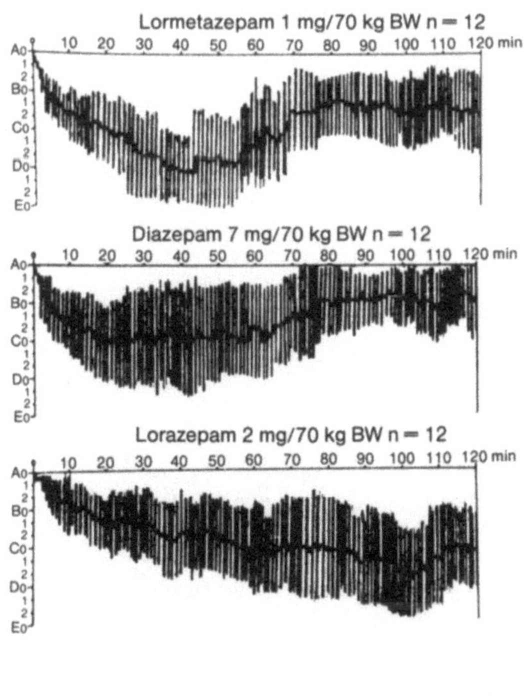


**Fig. 2.** Dose-effect relationship after lormetazepam, diazepam and lorazepam in 36 subjects (12 per group) in a randomized prospective study (double-blind). The vigilosomnogram showed the slightest standard deviation after lormetazepam 1 mg/70 kg BW. $A_0$–$E_0$: different vigilosomnogram stages

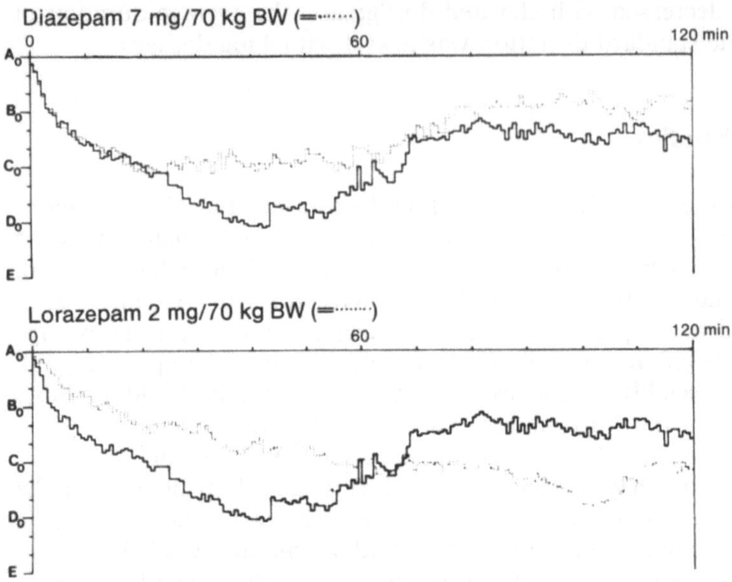


**Fig. 3.** A comparison of the mean vigilosomnograms (cf. Fig. 2). *Top:* lormetazepam 1 mg/70 kg BW (*continuous line*) and diazepam 7 mg/70 kg BW (*dotted line*). *Bottom:* lormetazepam 1 mg/70 kg BW (*continuous line*) and lorazepam 2 mg (*dotted line*). The sleep stages between the 25th and 60th min were shown to be deeper after lormetazepam than under the reference substances. $A_0 - E_0$: different vigilosomnogram stages

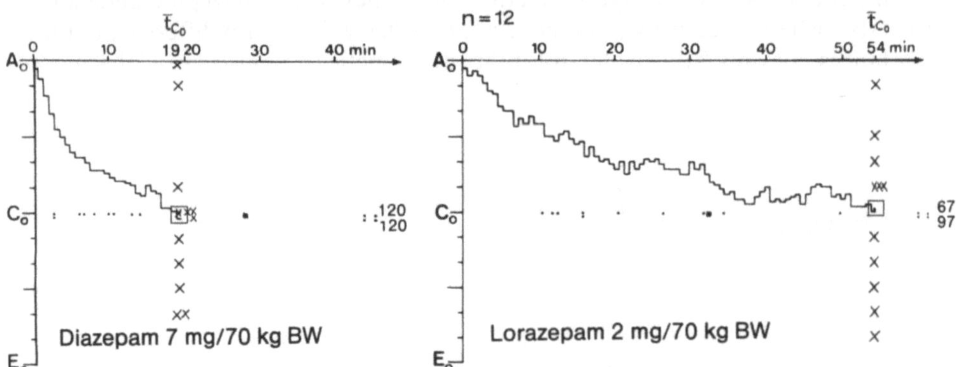


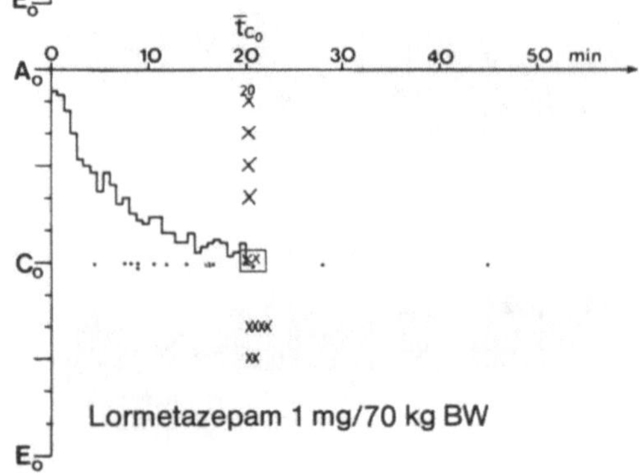


**Fig. 4** The latency to stage $C_0$ was reached about 20 min after the start of the injection of lormetazepam (SHF 312 BC) and diazepam, and about 50 min after the injection of lorazepam (see Fig. 2). Stage $C_0$ combined with an analgesic component is sufficient for anaesthesia. $A_0 - E_0$: different vigilosomnogram stages. ● Individual indices of vigilance at $\bar{t}_{C_0}$; ■ individual latencies to $C_0$; □ mean latency $\bar{t}_{C_0}$

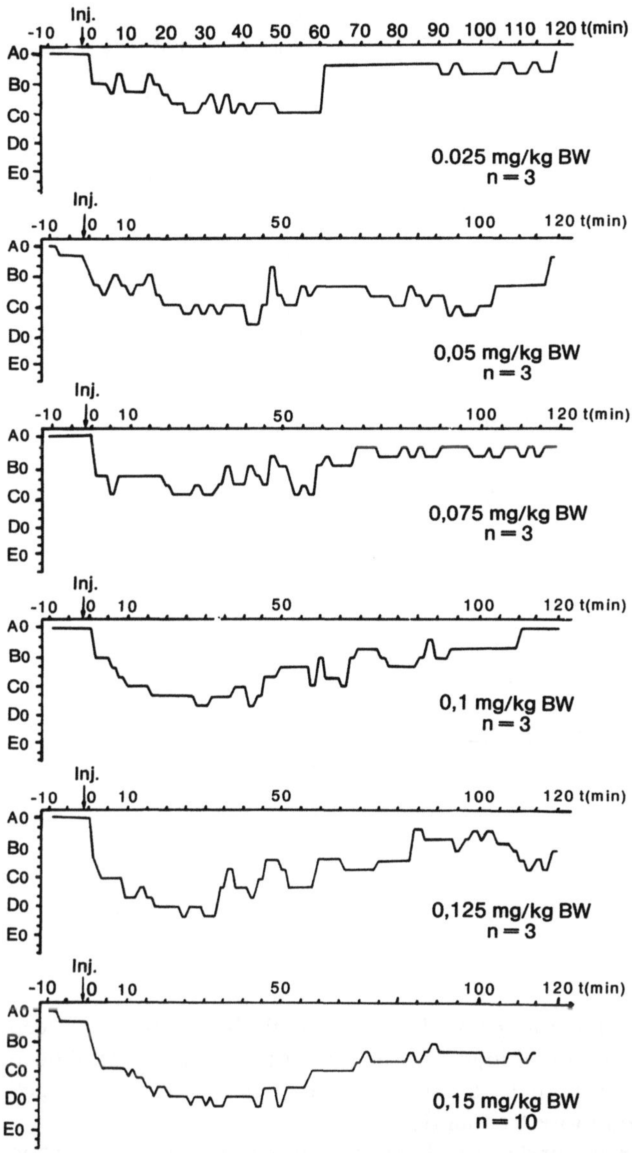


**Fig. 5.** Dose-effect relationships after midazolam. With doses from 0.1 mg/kg BW sufficient sleep stages ($C_0$) are attained up to the 60th min. $A_0$–$E_0$: different vigilosomnogram stages

dynamics. In order to obtain comparable vigilosomnographic results, it was first necessary to obtain dose-effect curves (Fig. 5).

Even the lowest dose of 0.025 mg/kg resulted in transient deep sleep. Increased doses resulted in a prolongation of the deep hypnotic state $C_0$ and more, lasting 60 to 100 min following the application of 0.15 mg of midazolam (Fig. 6).

Clinical observations on patients may have produced the impressions of fast sleep induction because of the absence of the lid reflex or other signs, but reproducible results which are statistically valid require a prospective, controlled study monitored by EEG under standard and comparable conditions (Grote et al. 1980).

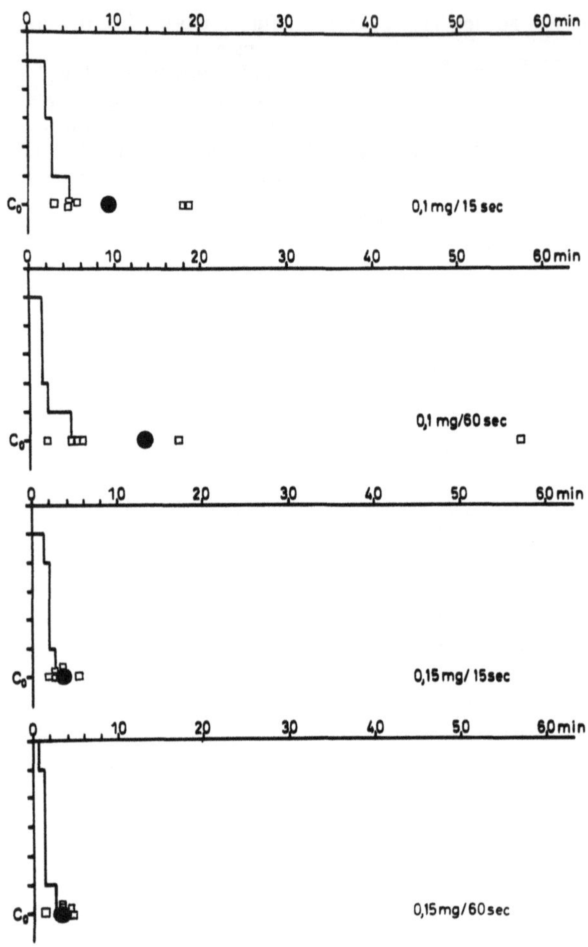


**Fig. 6.** In a randomized, prospective study (24 subjects) the latency (attainment of stage $C_0$) was recorded dependent on the injection time and dose of midazolam. Stage $C_0$ is apparent within 1–2 min after injection of 0.15 mg/kg BW midazolam with an injection time of 15 and 60 s. After 0.1 mg/kg BW the latency is delayed. □ Individual attainment of stage $C_0$; ● mean value

It is also possible to correlate the speed of injection with the dynamics of sleep induction, i.e. the shorter the time of injection the more quickly the stage of deep sleep is reached. Side-effects such as a fall in blood pressure and prolonged periods of apnoea are noted more frequently.

In this clinical experiment under EEG control, the heart and circulation (intra-arterial blood pressure) and respiration (capnography) were monitored enabling us to ascertain optimal dosage and duration of injection. These results are applicable to clinical conditions. Midazolam, after the dose-effect relationship had been established, was administered in two different dosages and speeds of injection. Four groups of six subjects each, randomly distributed, received either 0.1 mg/kg body weight within 15 or 60 s, or 0.15 mg/kg body weight also within 15 or 60 s.

Both latency and median onset of sleep time decreased with increased dosage, so that adequate depth of sleep was reached in a few minutes. On the basis of these observations, midazolam must be considered as one of the most potent benzodiazepines. There is evidence of sedation even up to hypnosis already after minimal doses.

## 3 Combined Studies Using Anaesthesia

To exclude subjective influences, we used the following methods of anaesthesia in 12 subjects, following a random double cross-over design: Induction with propanidid after intubation under pancuronium and controlled respiration with nitrous oxide/oxygen; in the 15th minute after induction either 15 mg droperidol or 2 mg lormetazepam were given i.v. Each subject was anaesthetized twice for two hours on each occasion, so that altogether 24 vigilosomnograms were completed.

According to the EEG-based vigilosomnograms (average values and standard deviations, see Fig. 7), the lormetazepam/oxygen/nitrous oxide combination produced an additive increase in the depth of the hypnotic effect. After droperidol the specific nitrous oxide component of the depth of sleep at $B_0$ stage (from the 10th to the 15th minute this was well marked) was not exceeded. For statistical evaluation corresponding intervals were determined and the respective plans com-

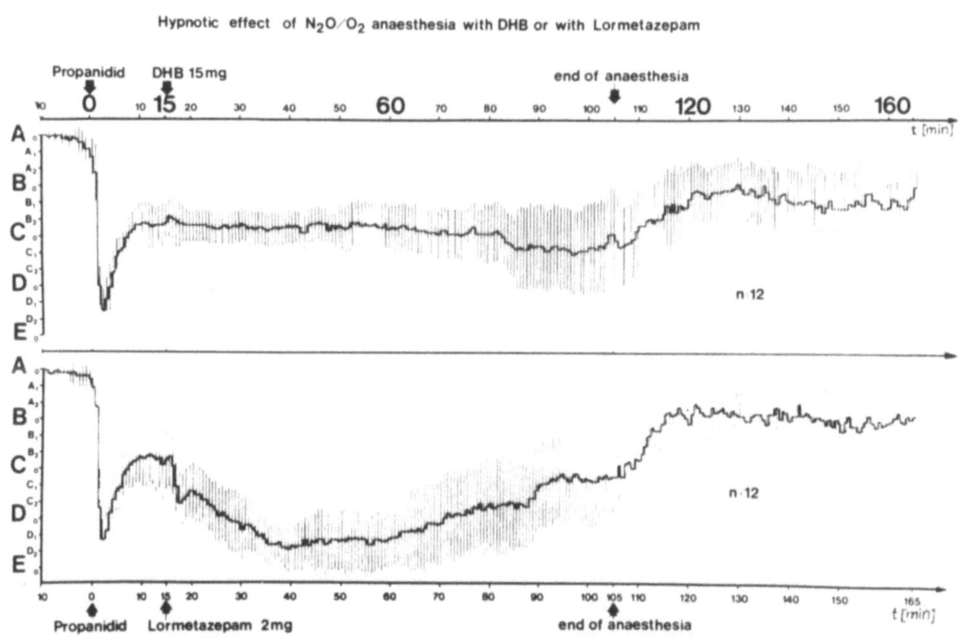


**Fig. 7.** Anaesthesia was induced by intravenous application of propanidid followed by intubation with pancuronium under nitrous oxide. Droperidol (DHB) and lormetazepam were applied in the 15th minute in an attempt to maintain the anaesthesia (randomized, prospective, 12 subjects per group with a crossover design). Droperidol had no influence on the nitrous oxide anaesthesia. Deep sleep was induced immediately after the injection of lormetazepam, reaching stage $E_0$. $A_0-E_0$: different vigilosomnogram stages

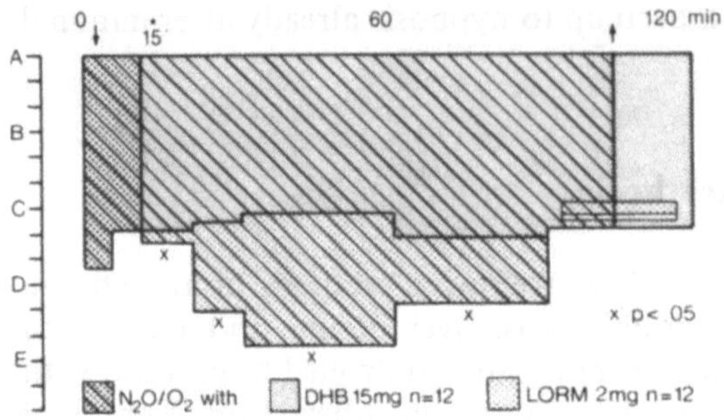


**Fig. 8.** A summary of vigilosomnograms (see Fig. 7) in large time spans. Crosses indicate significant differences between the two treatment groups

pared. The differences in depth of sleep between droperidol and lormetazepam are significant at the $p < 0.05$ level (Fig. 8). It is known from earlier experiments that such deep stages of sleep cannot be attained after 2 mg lormetazepam without basal narcosis (reaching the $C_0$ stage at most) as are obtained with the combination lormetazepam/nitrous oxide/oxygen.

These results confirm the findings in animal experiments by a group of workers under Stumpf who postulated supra-additive effects of benzodiazepines as opposed to droperidol (Stumpf et al. 1975).

## 4 Psychometric Tests and Appraisal

After these comparative investigations of anaesthetics, psychometric tests in the form of lists of symptoms were particularly informative. Psychic changes occurred up to 72 h. The subjects felt constricted, under some circumstances with a strong feeling of unrest, vegetative abnormalities, and some with Parkinsonian symptoms. After benzodiazepines all subjects recovered quickly whereas none wished to undergo anaesthesia with droperidol again.

It must be remembered that droperidol – a highly effective neuroleptic with a long duration of action (24 to 48 h) – is also used in premedication for the purpose of sedation and relief of anxiety. In this connection we would question the use of butyrophenones as adjuvants in anaesthesia on the basis of the side-effects established recently and 16 years ago or, at least, recommend that their dosage be greatly reduced.

From an anaesthesiological point of view controllability of a substance is determined by the duration of effect (short- or long-acting) and by the depth of sleep (light or deep states) achieved.

By these criteria midazolam appears to exhibit good controllability with regard to duration, but not in terms of depth of sleep, since it follows the "all-or-nothing" rule, even with 0.1 mg/kg both of intravenous or intramuscular injection. Lormetazepam, on the other hand, allows good controllability of depth of sleep from tranquillity via sedation to hypnosis, but the duration of effect is less well controllable in that patients remain lightly asleep even after 2 hours.

Flunitrazepam in our opinion takes an intermediate position between lormetazepam and lorazepam.

*Concept of Controlling Anaesthesia*

1) With respect to duration – short/long term
2) With respect to sleep depth – light/deep sleep stages.

Midazolam: Good steerability with respect to duration; not as good with respect to desired depth of sleep since with i.v. and i.m. application of 0.05 mg/kg body weight deep sleep stages occur.

Lormetazepam: Good steerability with respect to desired sleep depth (tranquillizing, sedative, hypnotic); not steerable with respect to duration, as light sleep stages can be seen after 2 h.

Flunitrazepam: Midposition between lormetazepam and lorazepam.

## 5 Experience with Benzodiazepine Antagonists

The development of benzodiazepine antagonists marked a milestone in so-called benzodiazepine anaesthesia. The first results were announced in Cardiff.

Möhler and Okada (1977) found that the benzodiazepines are bound to discrete receptors on the membranes of the neurones in the CNS. The results of investigations into the displacement of benzodiazepines from their receptors led Hoffmann-La Roche to the synthesis of benzodiazepine antagonists. One of the antagonists, an imidazodiazepine, has shown low toxicity in animal studies and blocks the action of several benzodiazepines.

We studied these antagonists in a preliminary experimental clinical trial (Table 1). Six subjects were studied. Each received the antagonist Ro 15-1788 only, the antagonist and flunitrazepam 5 min later, or flunitrazepam and than Ro 15-1788 5 min later. EEG, ECG, cardiovascular indices and breathing were measured continously for 130 min. The subjects who received only the antagonist remained awake throughout the study (Doenicke et al. 1982).

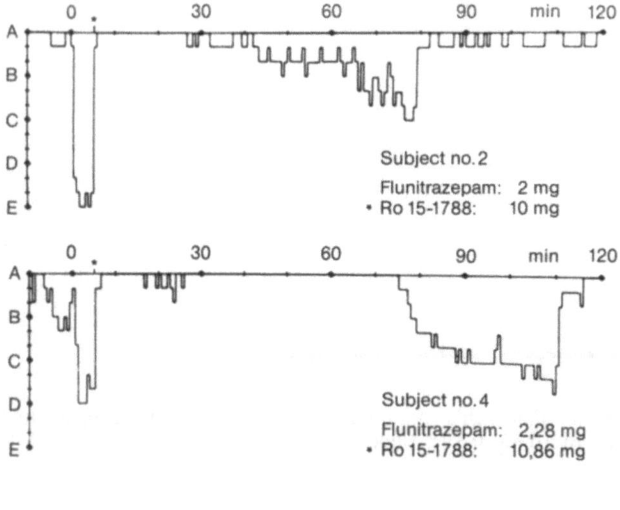


**Fig. 9.** Vigilosomnograms of subjects 2 and 4. Flunitrazepam was injected 5 min prior to the benzodiazepine antagonist. Ro 15-1788 had an immediate antagonistic action. *A–E*: different vigilosomnogram stages

**Table 1.** Protocol of the pilot study. The benzodiazepine antagonist Ro 15-1788 was injected 2 × prior to placebo (zero), 2 × prior to flunitrazepam (0.03 mg/kg BW), 2 × 5 min after flunitrazepam (0.03 mg/kg BW)

*Schedule*

| Minutes: | − 10′ | 0′ | 5′ | 120′ |
|---|---|---|---|---|
| EEG | ——— | ——— | ——— | → // |
| ECG | ——— | ——— | ——— | → // |
| Blood pressure | ——— | ——— | ——— | → // |
| Respiration | ——— | ——— | ——— | → // |
| Psychological testing | * | | | // * * |

| Subjects: | | | |
|---|---|---|---|
| No.: | 1 | Ro 15-1788 Dose: 10 mg | NaCl 10 ml |
| | 7 | Ro 15-1788 Dose: 15 mg | NaCl 10 ml |
| | 3 | Ro 15-1788 Dose: 10 mg | Flunitrazepam Dose: 2 mg |
| | 5 | Ro 15-1788 Dose: 10.86 mg | Flunitrazepam Dose: 2.28 mg |
| | 2 | Flunitrazepam Dose: 2 mg | Ro 15-1788 Dose: 10 mg |
| | 4 | Flunitrazepam Dose: 2.28 mg | Ro 15-1788 Dose: 10.86 mg |

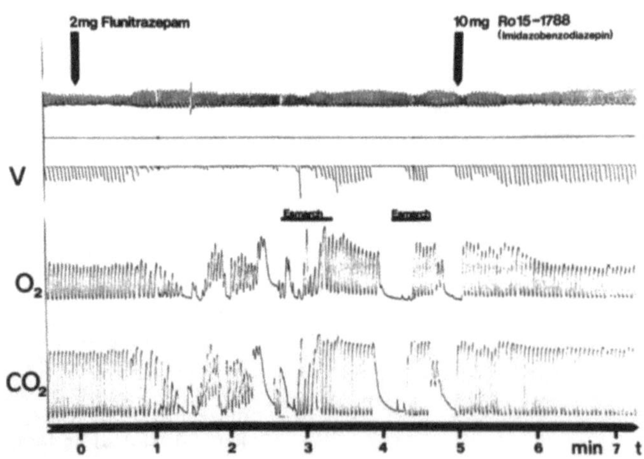


**Fig. 10.** Respiratory obstruction and Esmarch's manipulation after 2 mg flunitrazepam and immediate recovery after injection of 10 mg Ro 15-1788

**Table 2.** The schedule of the dose-effect relationship for the benzodiazepine antagonist, Ro-15-1788

*Schedule*

| | Flunitrazepam | | | | |
|---|---|---|---|---|---|
| | −10 min | −0− | Ro 15-1788<br>5 min | 120 min | 8 h |
| EEG, ECG<br>Blood pressure<br>Respiration | ********** | ******* | ********** | ********** | ****** |
| Psychometric tests | * | | | * | * |

*Dose* [mg/kg − 1]

| Subjects *n* | Flunitrazepam | Ro 15-1788 |
|---|---|---|
| 6 | 0.03 | 0.15 |
| 6 | 0.03 | 0.10 |
| 6 | 0.03 | 0.05 |

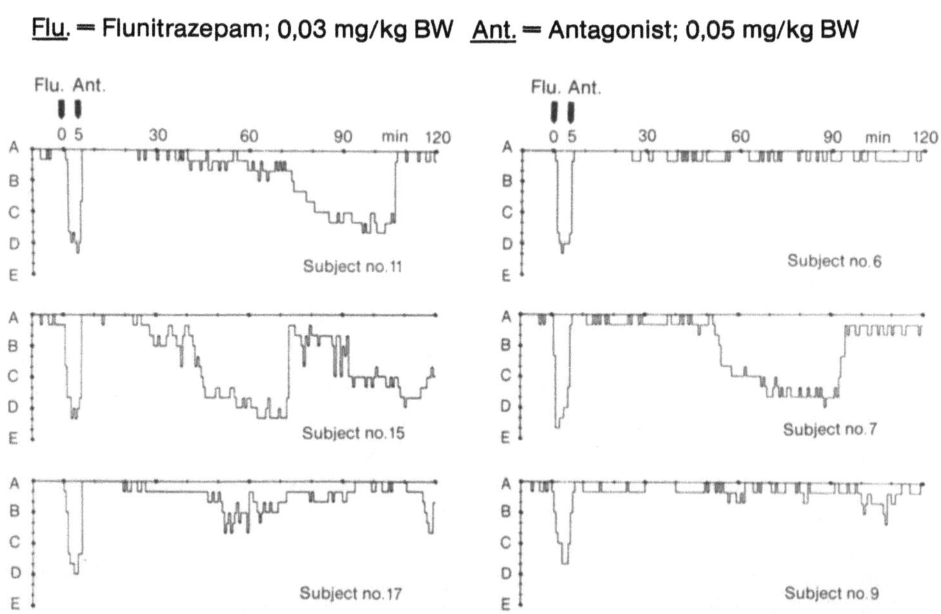


**Fig. 11.** Vigilosomnograms of six subjects after flunitrapezam 0.03 mg/kg BW. The smallest dose (0.05 mg/kg BW) of Ro 15-1788 is sufficient to distinctly antagonize the deep sleep induced by flunitrazepam. *A*–*E*: different vigilosomnogram stages

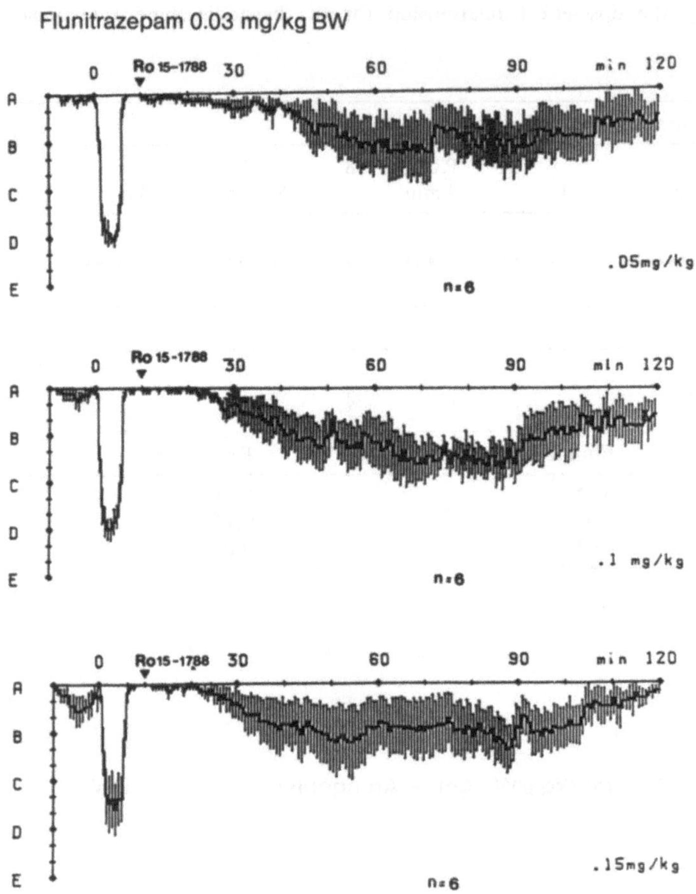


**Fig. 12.** The 3 mean vigilosomnograms from the study (Table 2 and Fig. 11) indicate that the antagonization is effective for 30–40 min. This period is followed by stages of slight fatigue. *A–E*: different vigilosomnogram stages

Five minutes after flunitrazepam, there was a return to the waking state ($D_0$-$E_0$) see vigilosomnogram, Fig. 9) in a few seconds, as a result of giving the antagonist. Following flunitrazepam, obstruction occurred several times (Fig. 10) so that Esmarch's manipulation had to be applied. Not only vigilance but also respiration became normal within a few seconds after injection of the antagonist.

If the antagonist was given 5 min before flunitrazepam was administered, the results were not so impressive. In one subject there were phases of sleep while another stayed awake for 130 min.

Since the subjects were observed in hospital for 12 h, we were able to establish that the four who had received flunitrazepam were sound asleep again 4 h after beginning the experiment. This observation points to a shorter half-life of the antagonist. It was possible, however, to interrupt this sleep by the application of arousal stimuli.

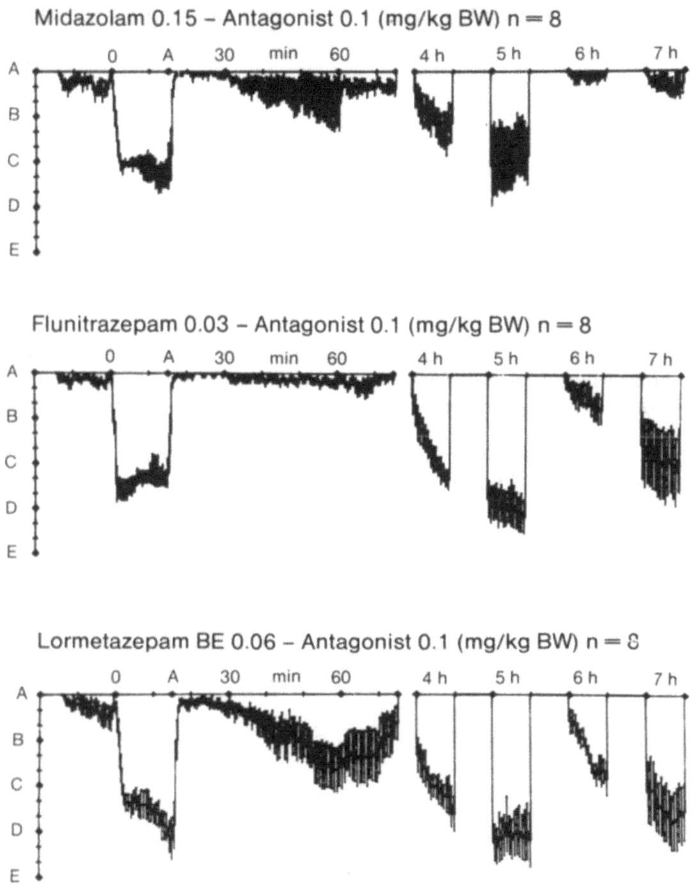


**Fig. 13.** Antagonization with Ro 15-1788 was also distinct after lormetazepam 0.06 mg/kg BW and midazolam 0.15 mg/kg BW. There were deep post-sleep stages for up to 7 h, both after lormetazepam and flunitrazepam. Subjects felt refreshed from the 6th hour after midazolam. *A – E*: different vigilosomnogram stages

After this pilot investigation another dose finding study was initiated (Table 2). 3 groups of 6 volunteers each were given flunitrazepam. The antagonist was applied in three different doses (0.15 mg/kg, 0.1 mg/kg, 0.075 mg/kg).

A prompt antagonism was noticed in all groups (Fig. 11). In some instances volunteers awakened within the first few seconds during the course of injection which requires 60 s. After 30 min, however, subjects fell asleep again.

A summary of the results obtained in these 18 volunteers is provided (Fig. 12). Volunteers were further monitored up till the evening. Between the 5th–8th hour subsequent to the application of the antagonist, they fell asleep once more.

In a third study undertaken during the last year, lormetazepam, flunitrazepam and midazolam were selected as agonists to test the antagonist in offsetting sleep and sedation (Fig. 13). An abrupt awakening was also evident following the administration of all three agonists. Post sleep phases, which were independent of the agonists' individual half-lives, were also observed in the following 8 h control phase.

## References

Doenicke A, Kugler J, Suttmann H, Grote B, Donner W (1980) Midazolam: Abhängigkeit der Schlaftiefe von Injektionszeit und Dosis. Anaesthesist 29:637

Doenicke A, Kugler J, Suttmann H, Ott H, Grote B (1981) New benzodiazepines. Excerpta Medica. Int Cong Series 538:722

Doenicke A, Suttmann H, Kugler J, Kapp W, Wolf R (1982) Pilot study of a benzodiazepine antagonist. Br J Anaesth 54:1183

Grote B, Doenicke A, Kugler J, Suttmann H, Laub M (1980) Midazolam: Dosisfindung mit Hilfe des Encephalogramms. Anaesthesist 29:635

Möhler H, Okada T (1977) Benzodiazepine receptor: demonstration in the central nervous system. Science 198:849

Stumpf Ch, Gogolak G, Huck S, Andics A (1975) Wirkung zentral dämpfender Pharmaka auf die Stickoxydul-Narkose. Anaesthesist 24:264

# Are Electroencephalographic and Psychomotor Measures Sensitive in Detecting Residual Sequelae of Benzodiazepine Hypnotics?

H. Ott[1]

**Contents**



**Abstract**

*Purpose:* The recent development of short-acting benzodiazepines without active metabolites calls for a differentiation between the hangover effects of long-acting (LBD) and short-acting (SBD) benzodiazepines, when used as nighttime sedatives. The question now arises as to which electrophysiological and psychometric tests can record these effects with the highest degree of sensitivity.

*Subjects and methods:* 35 healthy volunteers participated in 3 randomized double-blind placebo-controlled studies. In the first 2 studies the short-acting benzodiazepine (LORMetazepam 2 mg), the medium-acting BD (FLUNitrazepam 2 mg) and the long-acting BDs (FLURazepam 30 mg and DIAZepam 10 mg) were administered in single oral doses at bedtime. Hangover was measured in the morning hours prior to administration, and 12, 36, and either 60 h (first study) or 156 h (second study) p.a. The measurements included the pharmaco-EEG, particularly the relative power in the beta band; visual analogue scales for assessing the subjective quality of sleep, EWL-adjective check list; pegboard test and radioreceptor assay. In the third study, a single oral dose of LORM 2 mg was given and the acute sedative effects were measured by the Adaptive Pursuit Tracking Test, Pauli memory test, pegboard and Pursuit Rotor.

*Results:* The sleep-inducing properties of all BDs could be detected quite clearly on the first night p.a. Distinct hangover effects of LBD were apparent in the pegboard test and residual

1 Research Laboratories, Section Psychometrics, Schering AG, D-1000 Berlin 65, FRG

Psychopharmacology Supplementum 1
Editors: I. Hindmarch, H. Ott and T. Roth

effects in different beta frequency bands after the first and, to a lesser degree, second nights. Such effects were barely detectable after the SBD. The time course of the RRA plasma levels of LORM and FLUN corresponded well to that of behaviour. The correspondence for DIAZ was less clear.

The pharmaco-EEG proved to be the most sensitive measure of benzodiazepine effects, followed by continuous performance measures, such as the pursuit tracking test and driving simulator. Relatively low discriminability was observed with the discontinuous psychomotor tests, such as pegboard. These results have been interpreted within a concept of "activation theory" and it has been concluded that benzodiazepines more likely affect higher central nervous activities, such as the level of vigilance and attention, than simple activities, such as visuomotor performance.

**Key Words**

Adaptive Pursuit Tracking Test/Driving simulator/EWL-adjective check list/Hangover effects/ Flunitrazepam/Lormetazepam/Pauli memory test/Pegboard test/Pharmaco-EEG/Pursuit Rotor/Pursuit tracking test/Radioreceptor assay/Visual analogue scales.

## 1 Introduction

Ever since benzodiazepines first found clinical use as hypnotics, investigators in the field of psychopharmacology have been faced with the question of the intrinsic relationship between sleep, benzodiazepines and performance, the theme of this workshop (Randall 1961). Yet there is no simple answer. The reciprocity of completely different physiological conditions, i.e. sleep in an unconscious state and wakefulness with a high level of consciousness and activation, has first to be investigated and the different pharmacological profiles and pharmacodynamics of the benzodiazepines must be considered. One must also expect that, due to their varied nature, the methods employed in these pharmacopsychological areas, such as all-night EEG, performance tests and radioreceptor assay, can only yield limited correlations (Ott et al. 1982).

I have stated the critical considerations underlying the three empirical studies which were carried out in order to discover:

- whether the recently developed short-acting benzodiazepines induce nighttime sleep in the same way as the long-acting benzodiazepines,
- whether, after a single oral administration in the evening, they bring about hangover effects on the following day(s),
- whether certain methods, e.g. EEG, radioreceptor assay, Vienna Determination Apparatus, Pauli test, pegboard, questionnaires, driving simulator, Adaptive Pursuit Tracking Test etc., are more sensitive than other instruments in recording pharmacodynamic effects,
- whether the results can be fitted into a modern concept of activation theory with the areas "subvigilance", "attention" and "impulsion" and thereby interpreted in some meaningful relationship.

In order to answer these questions, three prospective experimental studies were carried out in young healthy subjects. The first two studies investigated hangover 12 hours and longer after administration, while the third study dealt with the acute effects of benzodiazepines on diverse behavioural measurements.

## 2 Residual Sequelae of Different Benzodiazepines

In the wake of the recent development of short-acting benzodiazepines without active metabolites, one has been prompted to examine whether the hangover effects of the long- and short-acting benzodiazepines can be differentiated when these are used as nighttime sedatives. The effects of the long-acting compounds, diazepam and flurazepam, of the medium-acting substance, flunitrazepam, and of the short-acting compound, lormetazepam, were assessed by the following methods:

- The pharmaco-EEG (Herrmann 1982), where the target variable was the frequency of beta waves which is known to be increased by benzodiazepines (Kugler et al. 1980). The 5-min resting EEG was recorded from the $A_2$-$O_2$ lead according to the international 10–20 system and the power spectrum was analysed. Changes in total power and relative power of different frequency bands were measured.
- Performance on the pegboard test, where the target variable was the time taken to remove 25 metal pins from the left side of a panel into a row of holes on the right side (Ott et al. 1982).
- A subjective assessment of inner states as measured with the EWL mood scale (Eigenschaftswörter-Liste; Janke and Debus 1977) where the target variables were the factor scores for "fatigue", "inactivation" and "activation".
- A subjective assessment of sleep quality and morning freshness with 100 mm visual analogue scales as well as time-related estimates of sleep latency, sleep duration etc. (Ott et al. 1981).
- Plasma levels of these compounds, assessed by the radioreceptor assay (RRA) as described recently (Dorow et al. 1982a).

### 2.1 Subjects and Design

23 healthy male volunteers, aged between 20 and 40 years, participated in the 2 randomized studies. The study design was double-blind crossover and placebo controlled with 2–3 weeks' washout phases.

#### *2.1.1 Substances and dosages*

In the first study, 30 mg flurazepam, 2 mg lormetazepam or placebo were administered to 15 subjects in single oral doses at bedtime. In the second study, 10 mg diazepam, 2 mg flunitrazepam, 2 mg lormetazepam or placebo were likewise administered orally to 8 subjects at bedtime. The dosages in both studies met with the dosage recommendations of the manufacturers, except in the case of lormetazepam which was administered in twice the recommended dose.

Hangover was measured with the 5-min pharmaco-EEG and the above-mentioned test battery prior to ingestion and 12, 36, 60 h (study 1) or 156 h (study 2) after administration. At the same times blood samples were taken for the radioreceptor assay.

*2.1.2 Biometrics*

All test parameters in the results recorded at the above-mentioned measurements were subjected to 3-factorial analyses of variance. If multiple comparisons were deemed necessary, then Tukey follow-up tests were applied, comparing the active compounds to placebo, so as to evaluate the medical and psychological significance of differences between the treatment groups. $p < 0.05$ was taken as the decision level and differences at the $p < 0.10$ level were interpreted as "tendencies".

## 2.2 Results

*2.2.1 Pharmaco-EEG*

The results of the first study in 15 subjects (Fig. 1) indicate that the proportion of the total beta band (12.5–30 Hz) in the placebo group did not change during any of the 4 measurement days. Flurazepam, on the other hand, significantly increased the beta power on the first, second and third days p.a ($p < 0.05$). Lormetazepam altered slightly, but not significantly, the beta-band proportion, yet its action did not essentially differ from that of placebo.

Figure 2 shows the results of the second study with 8 male volunteers. In this study lormetazepam did not significantly alter the beta activity when compared with placebo. Flunitrazepam, on the other hand, significantly increased the proportion of beta activity at 12 and 36 h after administration ($p < 0.05$ and $p < 0.10$). Diazepam also had an effect similar to that of flunitrazepam, but only at 12 h p.a. ($p < 0.05$). Dorow et al. (1982a) showed that the elimination half-lives for benzodiazepine-like activities after lormetazepam, flunitrazepam and diazepam, expressed in terms of lormetazepam binding equivalents, are about 10, 23 and 63 h respectively. Benzodiazepine binding equivalents after flurazepam are eliminated with a half-life of about 71 h (Dorow et al. 1982b).

*2.2.2 Pharmaco-EEG and Radioreceptor Assay*

Figure 3 shows how the time courses of the various substance concentrations in plasma correlate with the EEG activity in general, and with the beta bands in particular. The left and right ordinates represent the proportion of the beta band (12.5–30 Hz) and the lormetazepam binding equivalents (log scale) respectively. Since placebo is not an active compound, all values are below the detection limit. In the case of diazepam, the correspondence between the two factors is not particularly good. The drop in plasma concentration of diazepam observed between 36 and 156 h p.a. was not accompanied by a change in the beta-band fraction. The correspondence for flunitrazepam and lormetazepam, on the other hand, is rather good. The somewhat more persistent EEG effects of flunitrazepam may reflect its longer half-life and also the action of its active metabolites, i.e. the 7-amino derivative and N-desmethyl derivative.

Under treatment with lormetazepam, the rapid fall in plasma levels during the night had no effect on the beta-band recordings the next morning.

The increase in beta frequencies under treatment with benzodiazepines – also referred to as beta activators – is an established phenomenon (Kugler et al. 1980).

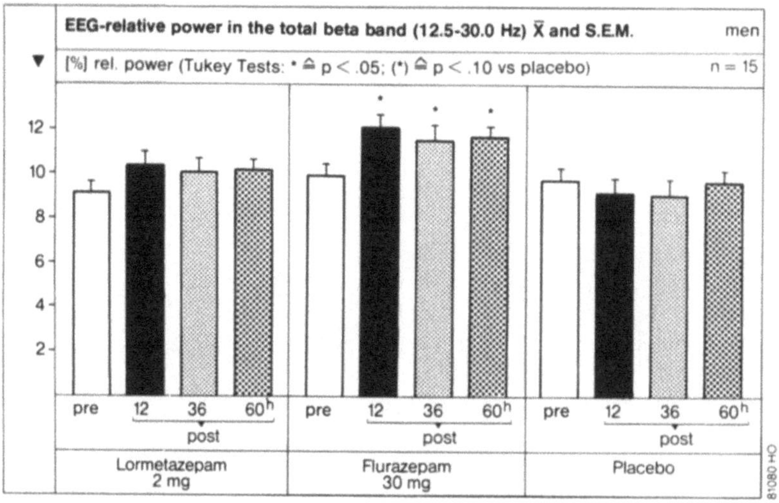


**Fig. 1.** Flurazepam induced a hangover effect in the total $\beta$-band 12, 36 and 60 h after single oral application, whereas lormetazepam and placebo did not show any change (study 1)

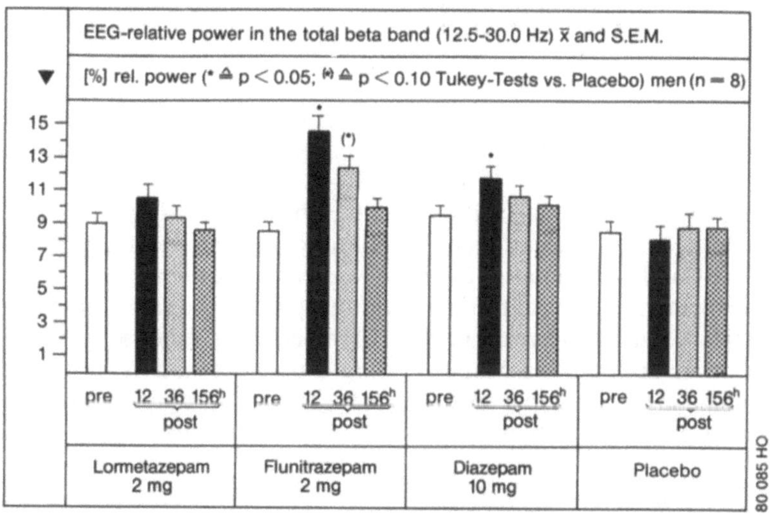


**Fig. 2.** Flunitrazepam shows $\beta$-induction 12 and 36 h post single oral application, compared to the relatively unchanged values of lormetazepam, diazepam and placebo. The unaffected values of diazepam are unexpected in the light of long-acting metabolites (study 2)

According to Bente, this increase can be interpreted clinically as a slight drop in vigilance (subvigil stages; Bente 1979). Here we should like to take up this line of argumentation.

### *2.2.3 Pegboard Test*

The pegboard test was completed immediately after the EEG recordings. The results of the first study indicate that this task can normally be completed within

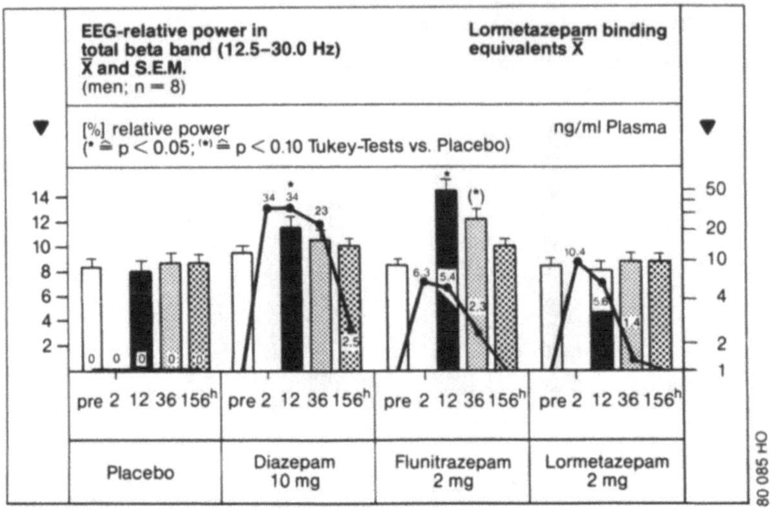


**Fig. 3.** The left and right ordinates represent the proportion of the $\beta$-band (12.5–30 Hz) and lormetazepam binding equivalents (log scale) respectively. Since placebo is not an active compound, all values are below the detection limit. The correspondence between changes in plasma level and beta fraction is rather good for lormetazepam and flunitrazepam, but not as strong as expected for diazepam (study 2)

about 35 s (see results for placebo in Fig. 4). It appears that lormetazepam had no perceptible effect on performance, whereas flurazepam significantly impaired performance 12 h p.a. ($p < 0.05$).

Figure 5 shows the results of the pegboard test in the second study combined with the radioreceptor assay. A clear, albeit not significant, increase in pegboard duration is apparent under diazepam 12 h p.a., whereas a significant ($p < 0.05$) impairment of performance is evident under flunitrazepam at the same measurement. The tendency towards a decrease ($p < 0.10$) in performance observed 36 h after ingestion of lormetazepam is a chance finding, a phenomenon of biological variability. In studies with a multiple crossover design, it is not unlikely that the values of some subjects will, by chance, fall outside the normal range.

### *2.2.4 Adjective Check List – "EWL"*

Figures 6, 7 and 8 offer the results deduced from 3 factors on the EWL adjective check list, "fatigue", "activation" and "inactivation". Under flurazepam, the feeling of tiredness (Fig. 6) and inactivation (Fig. 8) was significantly ($p < 0.05$) intensified in the morning on awakening (12 h p.a.), while the factor "activation" fell significantly ($p < 0.05$; Fig. 7). There were no biometrically significant changes in these factors of well-being under lormetazepam.

### *2.2.5 Subjective Rating of Sleep Quality*

The subjective ratings of sleep quality, measured on the basis of visual analogue scales, produced the following results: In the first study, a significant improvement ($p < 0.05$) was apparent in the assessment of sleep quality made by the 15

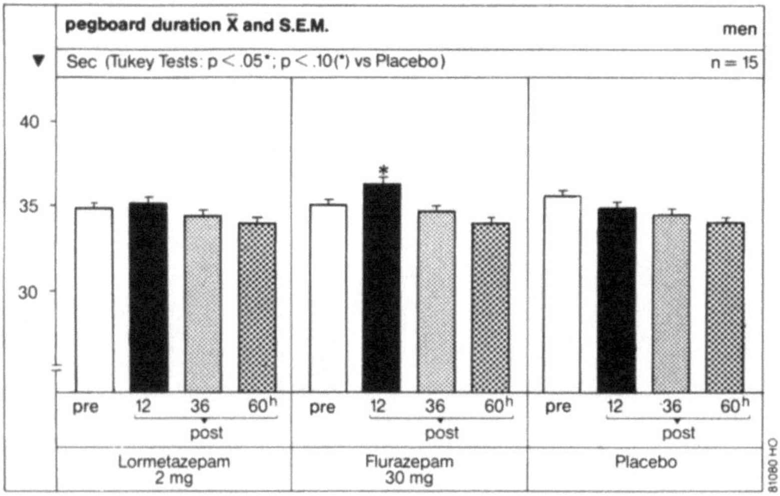


**Fig. 4.** In contrast to placebo and lormetazepam, flurazepam exerts an influence on the pegboard test 12 h p.a., which is interpreted as a psychomotor hangover effect (study 1)

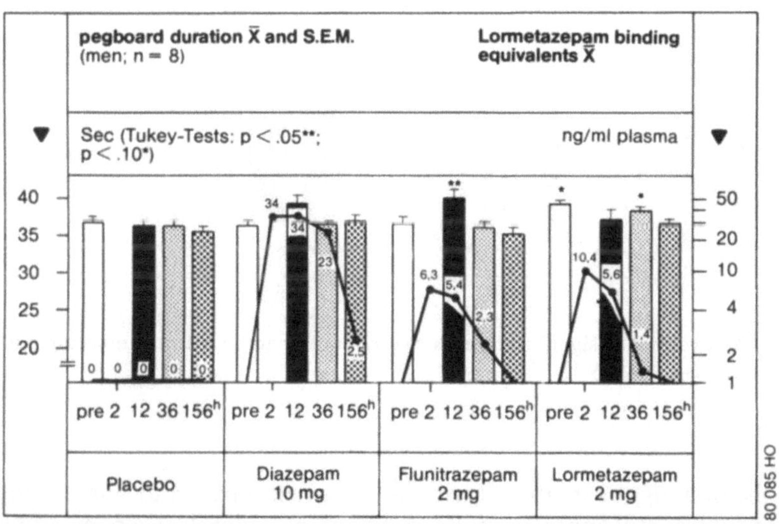


**Fig. 5.** Psychomotor hangover effects are induced by flunitrazepam 12 h p.a., whereas placebo and lormetazepam behave as if unaffected. Diazepam shows some insignificant tendencies of impaired motor performance. The correspondence between increase of pegboard duration (left ordinate) and plasma levels (right ordinate) are not as strong as expected for diazepam. The increase in pre- and 36 h-values of lormetazepam ($p < 0.10$) are attributed to biological variability (study 2)

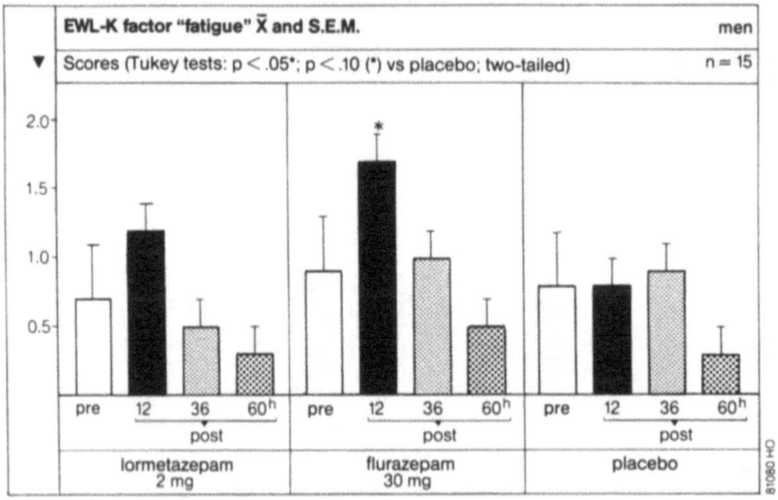


**Fig. 6.** In contrast to placebo and lormetazepam, flunitrazepam increased subjectively rated hangover, scored as factor "fatigue" of the "Eigenschaftswörter-Liste" 12 h p.a. (study 1)

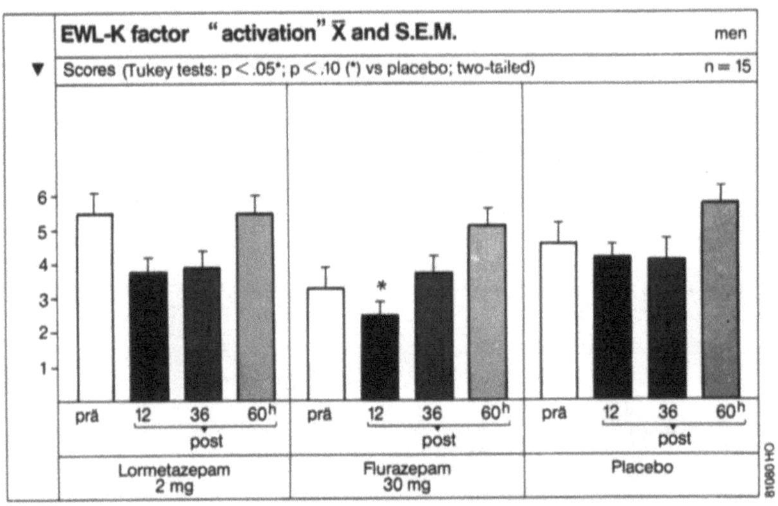


**Fig. 7.** The factor "activation" is significantly reduced by flurazepam in the next morning p.a. ("Eigenschaftswörter-Liste"; study 1)

subjects after the first night's treatment with both lormetazepam and flurazepam (Fig. 9). This effect was still apparent in the second night under flurazepam. After the second night's treatment with lormetazepam, a deterioration in sleep quality was assessed compared with the baseline level. This reduction was not significant and disappeared on the third day when the sleep-quality ratings approximately returned to baseline. The long-lasting effect of flurazepam, which was still apparent in the second night p.a., can be interpreted as hangover and, no doubt,

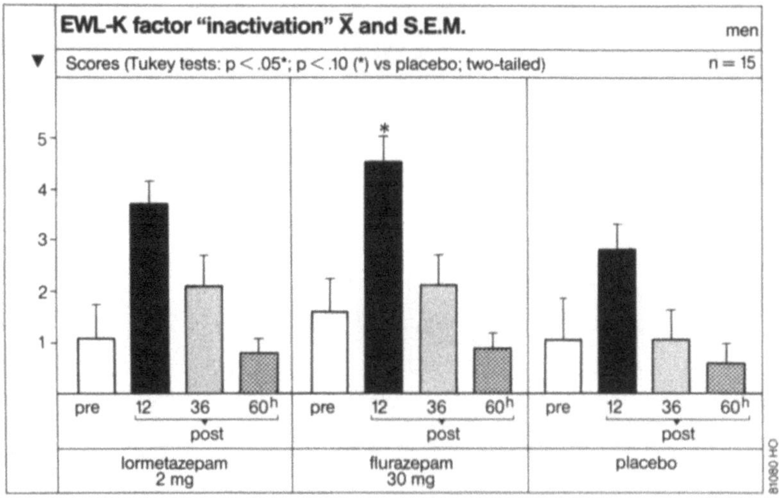


**Fig. 8.** The factor "inactivation", a subjectively evaluated inner state and scored on the "Eigenschaftswörter-Liste" is increased by flurazepam the next morning p.a. (study 1)

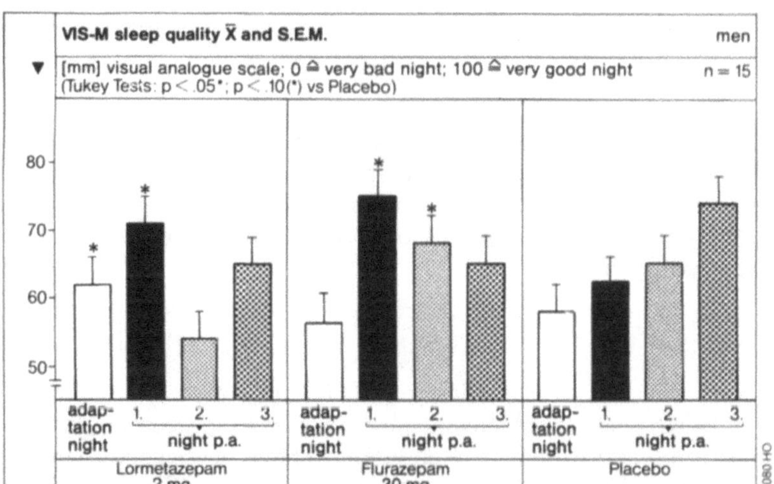


**Fig. 9.** In the first night, lormetazepam and flurazepam increase sleep quality assessed on the basis of visual analogue scales and compared to placebo. The high level of sleep quality in the 2nd night caused by flurazepam is interpreted as hangover after a single oral dose two nights before (study 1)

attributed to the long half-life of about 71 h of its main active metabolites, desalkylflurazepam (Dorow et al. 1982b).

Figure 10 shows the results of the second study measuring the effects of placebo, diazepam, flunitrazepam and lormetazepam on sleep quality in 8 subjects, again combined with the radioreceptor assay. As before, the effects of the drugs on sleep-quality ratings were compared with the concentration of the drugs in plasma.

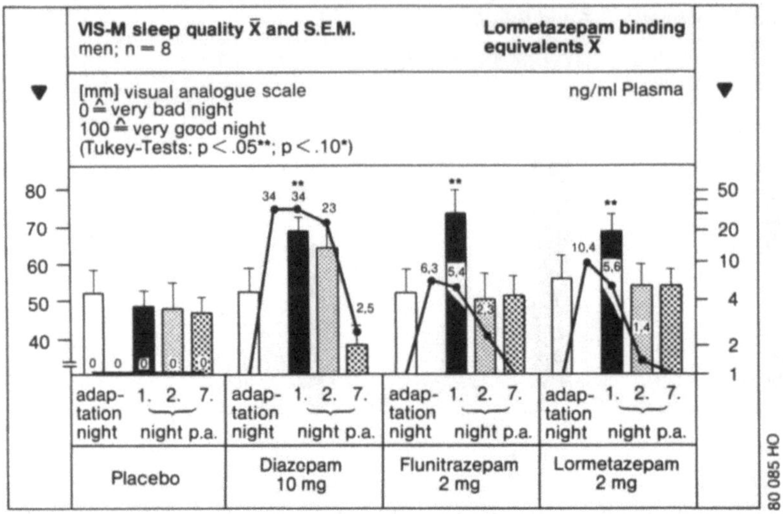


**Fig. 10.** In the first night, the three benzodiazepines, diazepam, flunitrazepam and lormetazepam, had a statistically significant and positive effect on sleep quality ratings. This effect was, however, absent in the second and seventh nights p.a. When comparing sleep quality with binding equivalents, the time course corresponds reasonably well for lormetazepam, but not as well as expected for diazepam (study 2)

In the first night, all 3 benzodiazepines had a statistically significant ($p < 0.05$) and positive effect on sleep-quality ratings. The same effect was no longer apparent in the second and seventh nights. When comparing sleep quality with binding equivalents, the time course corresponds reasonably well for lormetazepam, but not as well as expected for diazepam.

## 2.3 Discussion

Table 1 offers an overview of the statistical results from both studies. All compounds in the study were shown to have a positive effect on sleep quality, as experienced subjectively, and to reduce sleep latency. Thus the benzodiazepines proved to be good hypnotics with an adequate sleep-inducing effect. All drugs, with the exception of lormetazepam, increased beta-band activity for up to 3 days after ingestion. This can without doubt be seen as a drug-induced effect which, from a clinical point of view, is followed by a drop in daytime vigilance. Flurazepam and flunitrazepam also significantly reduced performance in the pegboard test. The performance decrements were also quite apparent under diazepam, and so this clearly must be interpreted as psychomotor hangover which, however, does not occur after lormetazepam. The subjects' sensation of fatigue and inactivation under flurazepam also adds weight to the objective proof of such decrements. Thus hangover after long-acting benzodiazepines was not only proved by objective psychomotor and physiological measurements, but also in the subjective sector and is, accordingly, of clinical importance. The results of both studies apparently confirm the working hypothesis that there is a correspondence be-

**Table 1.** Statistically significant hangover effects of different benzodiazepines on parameters of sleep, pharmaco-EEG and behaviour

| Parameter | | Substance (trade name) | | | | Interpretation |
|---|---|---|---|---|---|---|
| | | Flurazepam (Dalmadorm®) Day 1. 2. 3. | Diazepam (Valium®) Day 1. 2. 3./7. | Flunitrazepam (Rohypnol®) Day 1. 2. 3./7. | Lormetazepam (Noctamid®) Day 1. 2. 3./7. | |
| Pharmaco-kinetics | Half-life in hours (Radioreceptor assay) | ca. 71 | ca. 63 | ca. 23 | ca. 10 | Long, medium or short acting |
| Electro-physiology | Influence on beta frequency in Pharmaco EEG | – – – | – 0 0 | – (0) 0 | 0 0 0 0 | Hangover |
| Sleep induction | Influence on sleep latency (reduction in minutes) | 0 | + | + | + | Good sleep inducing effect (+); hangover (–) |
| | Influence on sleep quality (Visual analogue scales) | + – | + 0 | + 0 | + 0 | |
| Psychomotor activity | Influence on duration (pegboard test in minutes) | – 0 0 | 0 0 0 | – 0 0 | 0 (–) 0 0 | Hangover |
| Subjective well-being | Influence on fatigue | – 0 0 | Not measured | Not measured | 0 0 0 0 | Hangover |
| | Influence on inactivation | – 0 0 | Not measured | Not measured | 0 0 0 0 | Hangover |
| | Influence on activation | – 0 0 | Not measured | Not measured | 0 0 0 0 | Hangover |

*Explanation:*

0 No significant influence
+ Significant improvement ($p < 0.05$)
(+) Significant improvement ($p < 0.10$)
– Significant impairment ($p < 0.05$)
(–) Significant impairment ($p < 0.10$)

tween the time course of the active substance concentrations in plasma of long-, medium- and short-acting benzodiazepines and the corresponding hangover effects. There are, however, some inconsistencies, especially with diazepam, which require further investigation. Hypothetical explanations are presented in the following:

- The plasma concentrations of active substances and their active metabolites may not be a perfect reflection of the benzodiazepine ligand concentration at the specific benzodiazepine receptors in the brain.
- The long-lasting effect of active substance at the receptor could render the receptor insensitive, in the sense of possible tolerance development.
- Active metabolites, e.g. N-desmethyldiazepam, could exhibit an antagonistic effect (Elsass et al. 1980).
- Endogenous benzodiazepine receptor ligands could act in a counterregulative manner and thus absorb any clinical effect.

The different hangover effects of short-, medium- and long-acting benzodiazepines cannot be studied by pharmacokinetic methods alone. Electrophysiological and psychological tests, and subjective evaluations are necessary for an accurate differentiation between the actions of various benzodiazepines and for an assessment of their adequate clinical use.

In this respect, the pharmaco-EEG appears to be an impressively sensitive technique, this being reflected most prominently in changes of the beta frequencies.

## 3 Acute Benzodiazepine-Induced Performance Decrements Measured by Continuous and Discontinuous Psychomotor Tests

The electroencephalogram is, without doubt, a very sensitive method for recording pharmacodynamic effects and thus enables the investigator to trace slight residual effects of benzodiazepines in the elimination phases (see above). The EEG also has the advantage of a continuous recording. In contrast, the design of most psychological performance tests does not permit the continuous recording of performance during the execution of the designated tasks, e.g. the pegboard test as cited in the first study where 25 pegs had to be removed, one after the other, from holes on the left of the board and reinserted into holes on the right of the board. The test cannot record performance decrements or improvements during the hand's movement from left to right and right to left. The same applies to the reaction-time test and numerous other tests which can only record discontinuous responses to single stimuli. They can, in principle, only offer exemplary and accumulated values for relatively long test periods. Test devices which are employed to detect psychopharmacological effects, however, must be able to deal with the following factor: psychotropic substances are absorbed and eliminated in a continuous and non-linear fashion, often within relatively short periods, e.g. within minutes or even seconds in the case of intravenous hypnotics (for instance, etomidate, propanidid). Consequently, the field of psychopharmacology requires devices which can offer the continuous measurement of behavioural parameters and which can thus identify the important phases of kinetic action. An ideal solution in this respect is presented by measuring electrophysiological parameters, such as galvanic skin potential, ECG, actogram, and as earlier demonstrated, the electroencephalogram. Since the active participation of the subject or patient is not required when measuring these parameters, such methods can be employed independently of the level of vigilance, i.e. also during sleep, and the values can, in principle, be recorded continuously and simultaneously for as long as desired (e.g. over 24 h).

Psychomotor coordination performance, on the contrary, requires the active participation of the subject and is thus to a great extent dependent on physiological conditions, such as "fatigue", and psychological conditions, such as "motivation". Despite these restrictions, it seems appropriate to employ continuous visuomotor coordination tasks to measure drug effects (Nicholson et al. 1982). Such psychological tests are especially valuable, in that they have an immediate clinical face validity on the behavioural level, in contrast to electrophysiological methods, e.g. ECG, which can only detect impairments of the cardiac function. This point should be considered when dealing with CNS drugs which influence the total spectrum of human functions, especially activity and performance. A continuous visuomotor coordination task has been developed by Dr. Schaffler in Munich. It is the Adaptive Pursuit Tracking Test (APTT) and has been used by our work group in several psychopharmacological experiments.

### 3.1 Description of the APTT

The APTT is a complex method for testing fine and gross motor activity. A square target signal and a rectangular tracking signal are generated with different contrast onto a video monitor with a 39 cm screen. The aim of the test is to match the target with the tracking cursor using a joy stick. The degree of difficulty (size and speed of the cursor) is adapted to the number of errors and the performance capacity of the volunteer. In the present version the target moves back and forward across the screen oscillating horizontally. The better the volunteer tracks the target, the smaller the target and the cursor become, and the more quickly the target moves across the screen. The device records every deviation from the target signal cumulatively over a predetermined period and simultaneously records the momentary degree of difficulty (adaptivity) in arbitrary units. The mean level of the degree of difficulty corresponds to the mean level of adaptivity. The smaller the cumulative number of errors and the higher the degree of difficulty, the better is the tracking capacity of the subject.

### 3.2 Study Design

An experimental double-blind study with 12 young, healthy volunteers was performed in order to test the sensitivity of the APTT compared with other psychomotor performance tests. 6 of the subjects were given a single oral dose of 2 mg lormetazepam, and the other 6 received placebo. The study took place between 2 and 4 o'clock in the afternoon. The subjects had to complete a test battery before ingestion, and about 15, 40, 65, 90 and 115 min post administration. The

**Table 2.** Measurement times (min) of the psychomotor test battery completed prior to, and 5 times after a single oral dose of 2 mg lormetazepam

| | pre | ▼ Lormetazepam 2 mg | | | | |
|---|---|---|---|---|---|---|
| | | 1 | 2 | 3 | 4 | 5 post |
| Pauli memory | – 20 | 5 | 30 | 55 | 80 | 105 min |
| Pegboard | – 15 | 10 | 35 | 60 | 85 | 110 min |
| Pursuit rotor | – 10 | 15 | 40 | 65 | 90 | 115 min |
| Adaptive pursuit tracking | – 5 | 20 | 45 | 70 | 95 | 120 min |

actual testing times of the different psychometric tests are given in Table 2. The tests were attempted in the following order:

- Pauli test with memory span, duration 5 min
- Pegboard as described above, no time limit
- Pursuit rotor, duration 2 × 32 s
- APTT (mono) in the version described above, duration 5 min.

The Pauli performance test uses a modified principle of continuous addition according to Pauli (Pauli and Arnold 1951). The subject is expected to add together two single-figure numbers displayed in two windows, one above the other. The result, or second figure of the result (if above 9) is entered by the subject on a typewriter analogue located below the windows. The task can be made more difficult by darkening the upper window, and in its place the number displayed in the lower window has to be memorized for the next task. The Pauli test is thus an addition test which calls on the short-term memory. As soon as the subject types in his response, a new pair of numbers appears. The subject is instructed to work as accurately and as quickly as possible. The number of responses in 10 × 30 s intervals is recorded. Subjects normally attain a mean score of about 14 resolved tasks within a 30 s interval. The Pursuit rotor consists of a small 1 cm square light-spot which rotates around a circle at a constant speed (30 rotations per second). The subject holds a photosensitive pen with which he has to track the rotating light-spot. The time in which the pen deviates from the light-spot is recorded cumulatively in tenths of a second after 2 × 32 s intervals.

### 3.3 Results

Under placebo, performance became better in all four psychomotor tests, i.e. due to a learning process. The sedating action of lormetazepam was shown to interrupt this process. This was most evident in the APTT mono (Fig. 11): from the third measurement onwards ( = about 70 min p.a.) performance was almost twice as poor as under placebo. This also applied to the fourth and fifth measurements (about 95 and 120 min p.a.). The performance decrements under lormetazepam were further apparent, albeit less clearly, in the continuous tracking task of the Pursuit rotor (Fig. 14), whereby a trend towards deterioration was only identifiable at the 10% level (cf. Table 3) for measurement 4 (about 90 min p.a.).

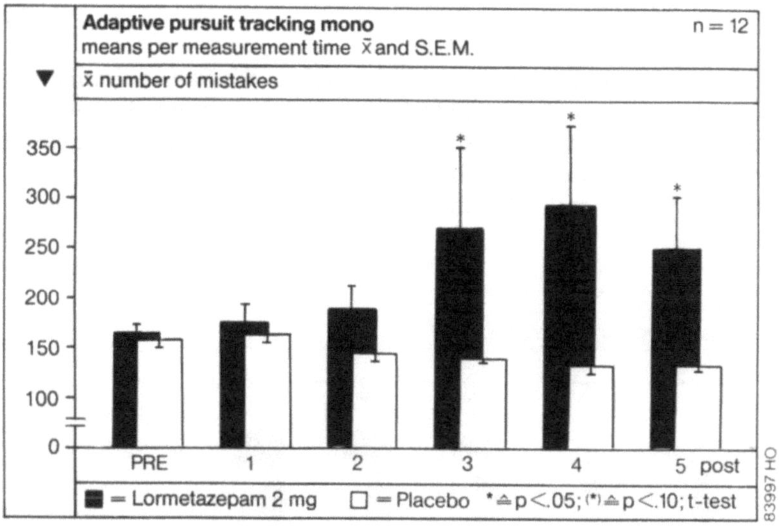


**Fig. 11.** Lormetazepam significantly impairs performance ($p < 0.05$; t-test) in the Adaptive Pursuit Tracking Test (mono) at measurement times 70, 95 and 120 min p.a. as compared with placebo. A learning effect is apparent for placebo

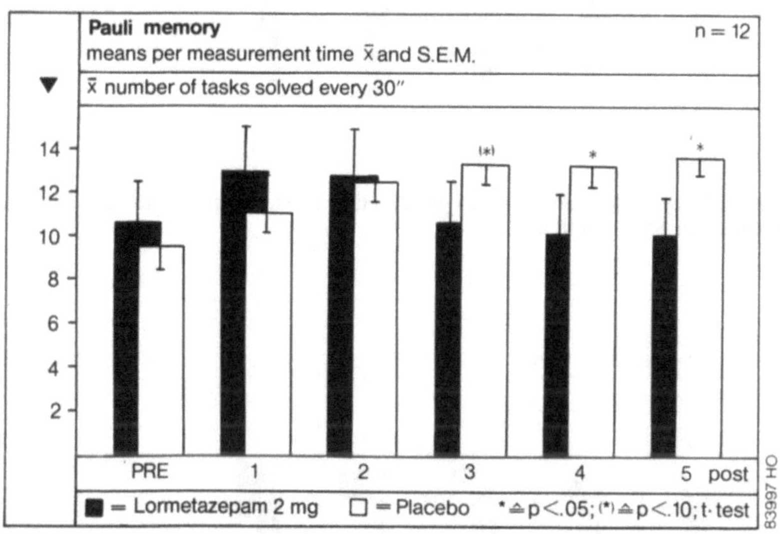


**Fig. 12.** Lormetazepam significantly ($p < 0.05$) reduces the number of responses in the Pauli memory test at measurement times 80 and 105 min. A learning process is evident for placebo

**Table 3.** Statistical results of psychomotor performance under acute dose of 2 mg lormetazepam; Differences post minus pre compared univariately to placebo; $n = 12$; double-blind, 2 independent groups; (+) ≙ $p < 0.10$; + ≙ $p < 0.05$

| | post 3 [min] | post 4 [min] | post 5 [min] |
|---|---|---|---|
| Pauli memory | 55: (+) | 80: + | 105: + |
| Pegboard | 60: 0 | 85: (+) | 110: (+) |
| Pursuit rotor | 65: + | 60: (+) | 115: + |
| Adapt. pursuit tracking test | 70: + | 95: + | 120: + |

Sedation was shown in the discontinuous cognitive task of the Pauli memory test (Fig. 12) to be tendential ($p < 0.10$; Table 3) from measurement 3 onwards, becoming distinct at measurements 4 and 5 (about 80 and 105 min p.a.; Table 3) with $p < 0.05$. In the discontinuous pegboard test the acute sedating action of lormetazepam was, at best, merely tendential ($p < 0.10$; cf. Fig. 13 and Table 3).

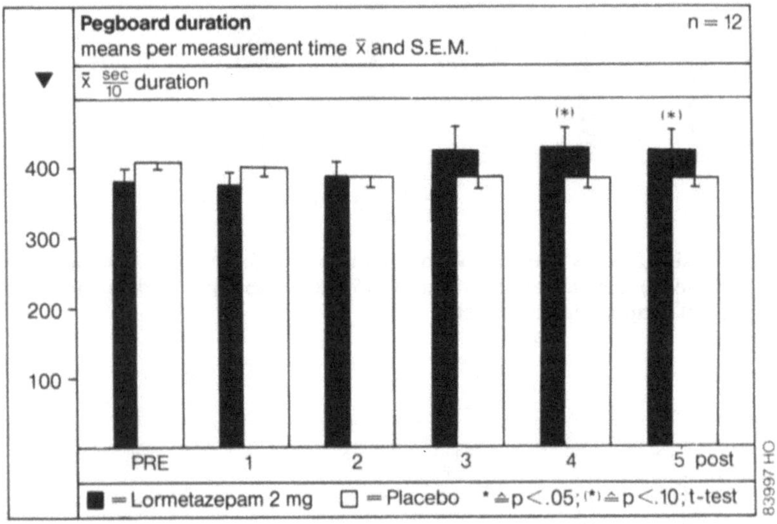


**Fig. 13.** There is a tendency for lormetazepam to prolong time needed to complete the pegboard test at measurement times 85 and 110 min p.a.

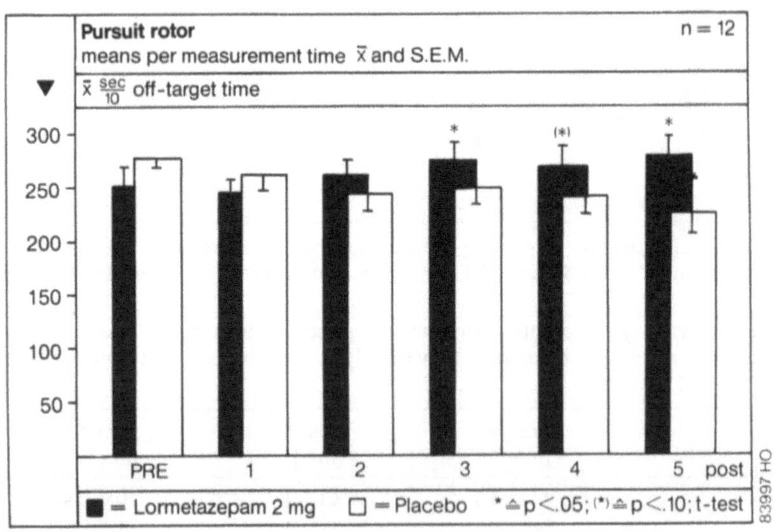


**Fig. 14.** The cumulative duration of errors on the Pursuit rotor is significantly prolonged by lormetazepam at measurement times 65 and 115 min p.a.

### 3.4 Discussion

The results of the empirical investigation of psychomotor tests on the basis of visuomotor coordination functions indicate that continuous measurement techniques, such as the Adaptive Pursuit Tracking Test and the Pursuit Rotor, are indeed more sensitive in recording a drop in performance than are the discontinuous visuomotor tasks, such as pegboard.

This finding is supported by the results of a study with the TS-2 driving simulator. In this double-blind study, the hangover effects were investigated in 26 subjects after an evening's intake of 1.5 mg lormetazepam, with and without alcohol (Willumeit et al. 1984). The set-up of the study included, along with the driving simulator, the APTT in the version described above, and the Vienna Determination Apparatus (WDG; Dr. Schuhfried, Mödling/Austria), which requires hand and foot reactions to different light and sound signals. The APTT recorded a noticeable reduction in performance under the combination of alcohol and lormetazepam ($p < 0.05$) which remained undetected by the driving simulator and the WDG. The correlation analysis revealed significant, moderately high correlations between the APTT and the WDG ($r = 0.41$; $p < 0.05$). No relevant correlations, however, could be established between the driving simulator and the WDG (see Table 4).

**Table 4.** Product moment correlation coefficients ($r$) between different psychomotor performance tests. The correlation coefficient between driving simulator and Adaptive Pursuit Tracking Test in relatively high (first arrow). A correlation between driving simulators and Vienna Determination Apparatus could not be found (second arrow)

| Test apparatus | | Driving simulator | Adaptive pursuit tracking | Vienna determination apparatus level 8 | | |
|---|---|---|---|---|---|---|
| | Parameter | Reaction time | Cumulative mistakes | Correct | Correct but delayed | Wrong |
| Driving simulator | Number minus mistakes | .04[a] ( .30)[b] | –.62 (–.57) ↑ | –.18 (–.11) ↑ | .02 (–.01) | .09 (.34) |
| | Reaction time | – | .27 (.01) | .08 (–.08) | –.08 (.04) | –.22 (.–26) |
| Adaptive pursuit tracking | Cumulative mistakes | – | – | –.10 (.01) | –.03 (.19) | .01 (.28) |
| Vienna determination apparatus level 8 | Correct | – | – | – | –.52 (–.49) | –.41 (–.29) |
| | Correct but delayed | – | – | – | – | .65 (.26) |

[a] Under Placebo
[b] Under Lormetazepam 1.5 mg; $n = 24$; $r > 0.41 = \zeta\,0.05/22$; $r > 0.35 = \zeta\,0.10/22$

According to empirical investigations within the framework of the activation theory (Duffy 1982), it would seem that the continuous psychomotor tasks, such as the APTT and driving simulator, record one common factor, the "attention factor", while the discontinuous tasks, such as the WDG and pegboard, record rather an "impulsion factor" (Ott et al. 1982).

In connection with the concept introduced in the above publication and the pharmacopsychological effects of benzodiazepines observed in this study, one can deduce that benzodiazepines influence vigilance and attention to a greater extent than psychomotor acceleration and speed. This deduction is supported by the findings of Kulikowski et al. (1984) who reported hangover effects of flurazepam in primarily cognitive tasks rather than in psychomotor reaction times. It is, of course, obvious to today's psychopharmacologists that this classification of benzodiazepine effects is dependent on the dosage, route of application, and length of time post application.

## 4 Conclusion

On appraising the results of the three empirical investigations, it would seem that a positive answer can be given to the questions drawn up at the very beginning.

Short-acting benzodiazepines improve nighttime sleep in the first night p.a. in the same way as the long-acting benzodiazepines, but the latter differ distinctly in their residual effects, depending on the half-life of the substance and its active metabolites. The electroencephalogram and the continuous psychomotor techniques, such as the tracking tests, are comparatively more sensitive in detecting these residual effects than are the discontinuous tasks, e.g. pegboard. This supports the concept of Ott et al. (1982) that benzodiazepines influence vigilance and attention rather than gross motor activity, i.e. benzodiazepines affect complex, rather than simple CNS-functions.

*Acknowledgement.* I should like to express my thanks to R. Dorow, K. Fichte, K. Hammer, U. Hippler, A. Rohloff and N. Sauerbrey for their assistance in the execution and evaluation of the study, and to H. Schermelleh-Solbrig and J. Horkulak for their kind assistance in the preparation of this manuscript. The Medicine Publishing Foundation is gratefully acknowledged for surrendering copyrights.

## References

Bente D (1979) Vigilance and Evaluation of Psychotropic Drug Effects on EEG. Pharmacopsychiat 12:137–147

Dorow RG, Seidler J, Schneider HH (1982a) A radioreceptor assay to study the affinity of benzodiazepines and their receptor binding activity in human plasma including their active metabolites. Br J Clin Pharmacol 13:561–565

Dorow RG, Hammer K, Ott H, Sauerbrey N (1982b) Correlation of benzodiazepine plasma levels with hangover effects as evaluated by radioreceptor assay, EEG and psychomotor performance. Paper presented at the Sixth European Congress of Sleep Research, Zurich

Duffy E (1972) Activation. In: Greenfield NS, Sternbach RA (eds) Handbook of psychophysiology. Holt, Rinehart and Winston, New York Chicago San Francisco Atlanta

Elsass P, Hendel J, Huidberg EF, Hansen T, Gymoese E, Rathje J (1980) Kinetics and neuropsychologic effects of IV diazepam in the presence and absence of its active N-desmethyl metabolite in humans. Psychopharmacology 70:307–312

Herrmann WM (ed) (1982) Electroencephalography in drug research. G Fischer, Stuttgart New York

Janke W, Debus G (1977) Eigenschaftswörterliste – Ein Verfahren zur Erfassung verschiedener Aspekte der Befindlichkeit (Version EWL-K). In: CIPS Collegium Internationale Psychiatrae Scalarum (eds) Internationale Skalen für Psychiatrie. Beltz Verlag, Weinheim

Kugler J, Doenicke A, Suttmann H, Laub M, Speth M, Woeller L (1980) Ein Vergleich der hypnotischen Effekte von Flunitrazepam und Lormetazepam. In: Doenicke A, Ott H (eds) Lormetazepam – Noctamid®. Springer, Berlin Heidelberg New York, pp 7.1–7.13

Kulikowski JJ, McGlone FF, Kranda K, Ott H (1984) Are the amplitudes of visual evoked potentials sensitive indices of hangover effects after repeated doses of benzodiazepines? In: Hindmarch I, Ott H, Roth T (eds) Sleep, benzodiazepines and performance: Experimental methodologies and research prospects. See this volume, pp 154–164

Nicholson AN, Stone BM (1982) Hypnotic activity and effect on performance of lormetazepam and camazepam-analogues of temazepam. Br J Clin Pharmacol 13:433–439

Ott H, Oswald I, Fichte K, Sastre M (1981) Visuelle Analogskalen zur Erfassung von Schlafqualität. VIS-A und VIS-M. In: CIPS Collegium Internationale Psychiatriae Scalarum (eds) Internationale Skalen für Psychiatrie. Beltz Verlag, Weinheim

Ott H, McDonald RJ, Fichte K, Herrmann WM (1982) Interpretation of correlations between EEG power spectra and psychological performance variables within the concepts of subvigilance, attention, and psychomotoric impulsion. In: Herrmann WM (ed) EEG in drug research. G Fischer, Stuttgart New York

Pauli R, Arnold W (1951) Der Pauli-Test. Eine sachgemäße Durchführung und Auswertung. München

Randall LO (1961) Pharmacology of chlordiazepoxide (Librium). Dis Nerv System XXII, Sec 2, Suppl, 7–15

Willumeit HP, Ott H, Neubert W (1984) Simulated car driving as a useful technique for the determination of residual effects and alcohol interaction after short- and long-acting benzodiazepines. In: Hindmarch I, Ott H, Roth T (eds) Sleep, benzodiazepines and performance: Experimental methodologies and research prospects. See this volume, pp 182–192

# Differential Effects of Benzodiazepines

# Are the Amplitudes of Visual Evoked Potentials Sensitive Indices of Hangover Effects After Repeated Doses of Benzodiazepines?

J. J. Kulikowski [1], F. F. McGlone [1], K. Kranda [2] and H. Ott [2]

**Contents**



**Abstract**

Here we compared the efficacy of two electrophysiological techniques in detecting hangover effects after repeated administration (five days) of benzodiazepines. Twelve hours after the last ingestion, possible effects on evoked potentials (EPs) of the long- and short-acting benzodiazepines, flurazepam and lormetazepam, were compared here with those of placebo under a double-blind experimental condition. The EPs were recorded from occipital and parietal sites during an active discrimination of two amoeboid shapes and passive viewing of sine-wave grating patterns turned on and off. In the former task, the subject was requested to make a selective response with respect to whether the two shapes appeared the same or different and his reaction times were simultaneously recorded. Neither benzodiazepine influenced the latencies of any of the sensory and late EP components. Flurazepam's long-acting metabolite, N-desalkylflurazepam, reduced the amplitudes of all the EP components suggesting a somewhat general mode of action. This was not the case for lormetazepam. N-desalkylflurazepam reduced the amplitudes of the occipital visual evoked potentials (VEPs) to sine-wave gratings to a greater extent than the amplitudes of the late parietal EPs to amoeboid shapes. This effect did not show any particular preference for either of the subsystems processing pattern and movement information. The amplitudes of the late EP components, such as N200 and P300 waves recorded from parietal sites, were reduced considerably more after flurazepam administration than their counterparts recorded from the occiput. This observation points to the possible existence of at least two separate sources of the N200-P300 complex with different affinities to the N-desalkylflurazepam. The flurazepam-induced amplitude reduction observed for VEPs to grat-

1 Visual Sciences Laboratory, Department of Ophthalmic Optics, UMIST, GB-Manchester, M6O 1QD
2 Research Laboratories, Section Psychometrics, Schering AG, D-1000 Berlin 65, FRG

Psychopharmacology Supplementum 1
Editors: I. Hindmarch, H. Ott and T. Roth

ings may reflect an attenuation in the detectability of both pattern and movement. The attenuation of the late EP amplitudes is possibly a function of several processes, one of which is conceivably the anxiolytic property of flurazepam which lowers the level of the activation state and this in turn is known to contribute to the amplitude size of the N200-P300 complex.

**Key Words**

Activation state/Anxiolytic property/Cognitive reaction times/Cortical neurons/Hippocampus/Lormetazepam/N-desalkylflurazepam/N200-P300 complex/Non-accumulating benzodiazepines.

## 1 Introduction

This study was undertaken to measure the hangover effects of benzodiazepines after repeated administration, and also to compare the efficacy of several techniques for detection of such effects. In the previous study, where we employed several techniques for investigation of potential hangover effects (Ciesielski et al. 1983), we observed great differences in their capacity for detecting benzodiazepine-induced effects. Since some techniques, such as the measurements of late components of evoked potentials (EPs) to amoeboid shapes, appeared promising we adopted a modified version of this procedure in this study. Other techniques, such as the measurements of flicker sensitivity and the critical flicker frequency (cff), confirmed our expectations as not being particularly well-suited for the measurement of hangover effects (see Besser 1967 for a time course of the cff after administration of diazepam; and Kranda 1982 for a theoretical treatment of this topic) and were therefore excluded. In their place we introduced measurements of sensory VEPs to sine-wave gratings, since patterns, unlike unstructured flashes of light, selectively activate cortical neurons. Grating stimuli presented in an on-off mode also offer the additional advantage of allowing the separation of pattern and movement components of the VEP (Kulikowski 1976, 1978a) where the amplitude of the pattern component can be reduced by the action of nitrous oxide (Kulikowski and Leisman 1973).

As in our previous investigation (Ciesielski et al. 1983) we administered lormetazepam and flurazepam to healthy subjects, but this time each drug and placebo was taken repeatedly on five successive nights. The rationale behind this aspect of the investigation was the attempt to assess the effects of chronic administration of two benzodiazepines on sensory and late EP components. Here we compared the potential effects of a long-acting benzodiazepine, flurazepam, whose active metabolite, N-desalkylflurazepam, has an average half-life of about 70 hours (ranging from 47 to 100 hours) with those of a short-acting benzodiazepine, lormetazepam, with an average half-life of about 10 hours (ranging from 8 to 14 hours) (see Greenblatt et al. 1981; Dorow et al. 1982; Kaplan and Jack 1983 for various half-life estimates). Since the metabolite of the former accumulates in the plasma after repeated administration, whereas the latter does not, we not only compared here the hangover effects of accumulating versus non-accumulating benzodiazepines, but also the effects of single dose (Ciesielski et al. 1983) versus repeated doses.

## 2 Methods

The two different techniques used for the investigation of benzodiazepine hangover effects were as follows:

a) Active discrimination response to pairs of amoeboid figures (Ciesielski 1982; Ciesielski et al. 1983) and a simultaneous recording of EPs.
b) Recording of VEPs elicited by passive viewing of sine-wave gratings turned on and off.

### 2.1 Amoeboid Shapes

These stimuli were essentially the same as those employed in the previous investigation (Ciesielski et al. 1983). In brief, the shapes whose luminance was 4 cd/m$^2$ were frontally projected on a tangent screen of about 2 cd/m$^2$ at a viewing distance of 172 cm. The stimulus pairs appeared for 60 ms 3 °45′ either to the right or to the left of the fixation point (a red LED) in the centre of the screen. Out of the total 32 pairs, 16 constituted similar shapes and the other 16 constituted different shapes. Both sequences, i.e. left-right and similar-different, were randomized. The centres of the shapes, each with a mean radius of about 38′ of arc, were 1.5 ° apart.

### 2.2 Sine-Wave Gratings

The gratings of vertical orientation were generated on the face of an oscilloscope (a modified D61a Telequipment). The screen with a green, P31 phosphor giving a mean luminance of about 20 cd/m$^2$ subtended 8 ° × 10 ° of arc at a viewing distance of 57.2 cm. Gratings of three different degrees of fineness were used on different occasions. Their spatial frequences were 2, 4 and 8 c/deg of the visual angle (i.e. each stripe subtended 30′, 15′ and 7.5′ of arc respectively). The gratings appeared once every 500 ms (2 Hz) for either 100 ms (condition 1) or for 250 ms (condition 2). The contrast ($C$) of the gratings, calculated according to the Michelson's formula:

$$C = (L_{max} - L_{min}) / (L_{max} + L_{min})$$

where $L_{max}$ and $L_{min}$ are the respective luminance maxima and minima of the bright and dark stripes of the grating pattern, was set to 0.3 (i.e. 30%). The screen was blank between two successive presentations, but its luminance equalled the mean luminance of the gratings.

### 2.3 Procedure

EPs and RTs were recorded on the sixth day (after five consecutive substance administrations) about 12 h after the last of the five capsules was ingested. Follow-up measurements undertaken at least 3 weeks after the last administration served as an additional control condition. Prior to the recording session the subjects were questioned briefly about their subjective feelings and the quality and length of their sleep.

a) The procedure for recording the responses to amoeboid shapes was similar to that employed previously (Ciesielski et al. 1983). The subject had to actively participate by pressing two response keys depending on whether the two peripherally presented shapes appeared to be the same or different. In contrast to the previous investigation, the subjects were instructed to maximalize their response accuracy rather than the speed of their response (Pfefferbaum et al. 1983).
b) The subjects were requested to view the gratings centrally so that their image covered all the central and paracentral portions of the visual field. Since only a passive observation was required of the subjects, the experimenter had to occasionally ascertain that the subjects maintained their central fixation and were reasonably alert. Breaks of about 2–3 min were introduced between successive averaging runs to reduce pattern-adaptation effects.

## 2.4 Recording Techniques

EPs were recorded with silver-silver chloride electrodes (resistance of about 1–5 kΩ) from $O_1$, $O_2$ and $P_3$, $P_4$ locations (according to the 10–20 system). Occipital and parietal locations were selected for recording EPs to amoeboid shapes, but only the two occipital locations ($O_1$ and $O_2$) were employed for recording VEPs to the grating patterns. The reference and grounding electrodes were positioned on the subject's earlobes and forehead respectively. The amoeboid EPs recorded from the occipital and parietal locations (Fig. 1 a) were only averaged for the hemispheres contralateral to the site of the presentation (i.e. $O_1$ and $P_3$ for right-field presentations, and $O_2$ and $P_4$ for left-field presentations). Sixteen presentations of amoeboid shapes to each half of the visual field sufficed for a satisfactory average, whereas at least 128 presentations of the grating patterns were required. The evoked signals were amplified with four identical Fylde electronic amplifiers whose filters had corner frequencies of 0.7 and 30 Hz and a 240 ms time constant.

## 2.5 Subjects

Twelve healthy males participated in, and completed the study. The subjects, whose average age and weight were 22 years and 70 kg respectively, were right-handed and had normal eyesight (6/9 or better with or without corrective refraction). They were instructed to abstain or at least reduce their alcohol, nicotine and caffeine intake to less than 5 oz alcohol, 30 cigarettes or equivalent weight of tobacco, and 15 cups of coffee per week, and to abstain from all these in the last 12 h prior to testing. The subjects, to our knowledge, did not receive any other medication or drugs during the period of the study.

## 2.6 The Substances and Their Administration

The two active substances were the benzodiazepines, flurazepam and lormetazepam, which are available on prescription in the U.K. Flurazepam is rapidly metabolized into an active substance, N-desalkylflurazepam, with a half-life of about 70 h, whereas lormetazepam has no known active metabolites and has a half-life of about only 10 h (Dorow et al. 1982). In order to ensure double-blind conditions, flurazepam 30 mg and lormetazepam 1 mg, and placebo were administered separately in capsules of identical appearance marked only with a code number. The code was broken after the investigation was completed. The experimental design was crossover where each subject received all three treatments in a different, but preset order. The subjects were instructed to swallow one capsule at bedtime on each of the five consecutive nights. Each of the three five-day periods, during which one of the three treatments was administered, was followed by a nine-day washout break before the next five-day period began, which meant that a full 14 days elapsed between successive tests.

## 3 Results

### 3.1 EPs and RTs to Amoeboid Shapes

The discrimination task adopted in this study elicits an EP waveform with two easily identifiable components (see also Ciesielski et al 1983). The two components in question, which we intend to use for analysing drug effects, are as follows: a negative wave with a latency (to its peak) of about 200 ms, referred to here as N200, and a positive wave with a latency exceeding 300 ms (P300). The peaks of these two waves are indicated by the arrows in Fig. 1 a. The amplitudes of these waves are, because of practical problems with establishing the baseline, defined here as the peak to trough, rather than the peak to baseline distance. The EPs in Fig. 1 illustrate typical results (close to the average of the 12 subjects) of one

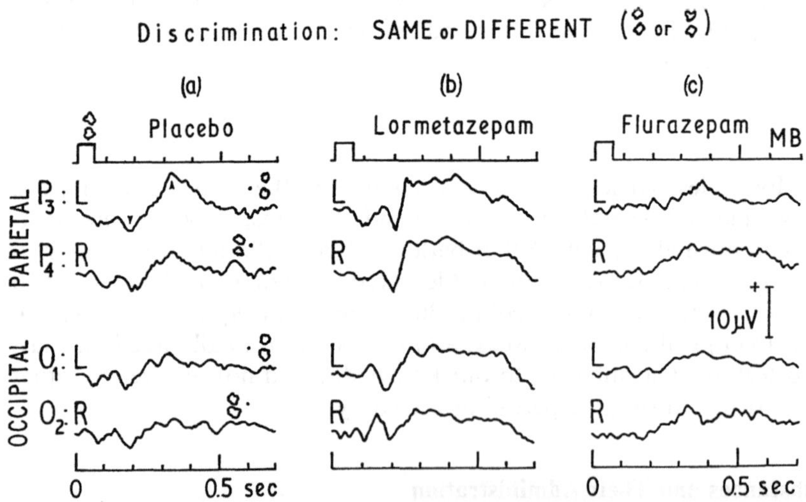


Fig. 1a–c. Evoked potentials to pairs of identical and different amoeboid figures presented at random for 60 ms. The averages (16 sweeps) represent EPs recorded always from the hemisphere contralateral to the site of the presentation. The three panels (**a**, **b** and **c**) show results measured about 12 h after the last administration of the respective substance. Subject M.B.

**Table 1.** Tabulated values of relative amplitudes (amplitude after drug/amplitude after placebo) of EPs to amoeboid shapes. The amplitudes of the N200 and P300 waves were measured in a peak-to-peak fashion. The amplitude averages and their standard errors are listed for 12 subjects

| Location | Parietal | | Occipital | |
|---|---|---|---|---|
| Drug \ Wave | P300 | N200 | P300 | N200 |
| Flurazepam | 0.69 ± 0.05 | 0.74 ± 0.06 | 0.81 ± 0.06 | 0.82 ± 0.09 |
| Lormetazepam | 0.99 ± 0.06 | 0.94 ± 0.08 | 1.00 ± 0.06 | 1.02 ± 0.07 |

subject. The only atypical aspect of this set of EPs is the unusually broad P300 wave observed after administering lormetazepam which serves here as an example of occasionally observed waveform variability observed in all conditions including placebo. Note, that only sixteen presentations are necessary in order to achieve a high signal to noise ratio and that the peripheral presentation reduced the early (sensory) components to a minimum. The most remarkable feature of Fig. 1 is the flurazepam-induced reduction of the N200 and P300 amplitudes. No such clear statement can be made about the latencies of the two waves since their amplitudes are reduced by flurazepam to such an extent that the position of the peaks becomes difficult to establish with a reasonable degree of confidence. Lormetazepam shows no effect on the latencies of either the parietal or occipital N200 and P300 waves. A potential lormetazepam effect on the latency of parietal P300 wave is, because of the flatness of the wave, difficult to establish.

The amplitudes of the N200 and P300 waves were determined for the other 11 subjects (total $N = 12$) in the same way. For the sake of facilitating a comparison of the potential drug effects on the amplitudes of the N200 and P300 waves, we listed in Table 1 relative amplitude ratios (i.e. amplitudes after drug/amplitudes after placebo). We further simplified the table containing the averages of all 12 subjects by merging ratios for left and right hemispheres (i.e. recordings from $P_3$ with those from $P_4$, and likewise $O_1$ with $O_2$). The single values in Table 1 are thus means of 12 subjects and both hemispheres with standard errors (SE). Lormetazepam appears to exercise no appreciable effect on the amplitudes of either the parietal or the occipital N200 and P300 waves. The effect of flurazepam on the amplitudes is, on the other hand, statistically significant and also somewhat more diverse, with at least two main courses of action.

1) Flurazepam is more effective in reducing the amplitudes of the N200 and P300 components recorded from the parietal rather than occipital locations.
2) Flurazepam appears to reduce the amplitude of the P300 more than it does the amplitude of the N200 wave. This is, however, observed only for waves recorded from the parietal locations.

### 3.2 Cognitive Reaction Times

In contrast to the previous study (Ciesielski et al. 1983), the subjects were this time encouraged to maintain a high level of accuracy rather than speed. Because of the trade-off between the speed and the accuracy of the response, it came as no surprise that the RTs were increased. The unexpected feature of this altered priority was the attenuation (compared to the previous study) of flurazepam effect on the RTs. Flurazepam increased the RTs by only about 5% (see Table 3) as opposed to about 12% reported by Ciesielski et al. (1983).

### 3.3 VEPs Elicited by Gratings

Passive viewing of the centre of the screen on which sine-wave gratings were turned on and off yields VEPs with components of short latencies (about 150 ms for the on response) and also of small amplitudes (see Fig. 2). The smaller amplitudes of the VEPs, compared with the EPs obtained during the discrimination task, and thus their unfavourable signal to noise ratio, requires a greater number of presentations ($N = 128$) in order to reliably identify the actual signal. Figure 2 shows VEPs to gratings of 2 and 8 c/deg presented for 250 ms twice per second (2 Hz). Both gratings activate the pattern- and movement-detecting structures in the brain but to a different degree. The 8 c/deg grating onset is believed to evoke predominantly pattern-related VEP responses, whereas the 2 c/deg grating elicits, in addition to the pattern-related, also a movement-related EP response. The relative contribution of gratings with various fineness to the pattern- and movement-specific neural structures is evaluated on the basis of the amplitude of the "off" wave (relative to that of the "on" wave), since the early components of the "off" wave contain only movement-related VEPs (Kulikowski 1978 b). The "on" wave, on the other hand, contains both pattern- and movement-related

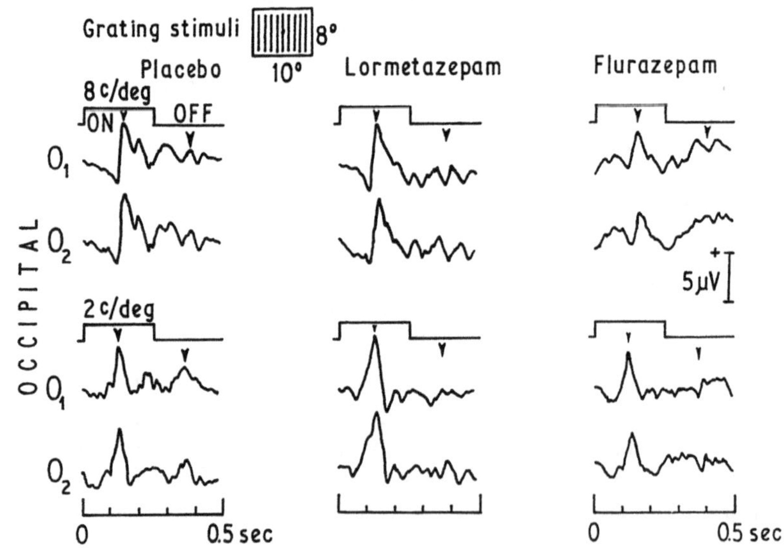


**Fig. 2.** Evoked potentials to sine-wave gratings turned on and off at the rate of 2 Hz. The gratings were viewed centrally and no active responses were required from the subjects. Recording was confined to the occipital region. The arrows indicate the peaks of the "on" responses and the presumed locations of their counterparts, the "off" responses which were assumed follow the "on" responses with a delay equal to the presentation of the stimulus, i.e. 250 ms. The two gratings had spatial frequencies of 2 and 8 c/deg.

**Table 2.** Tabulated values of relative amplitudes (amplitude after drug/amplitude after placebo) of EPs to sine-wave gratings of 8 and 2 c/deg. The sizes of the amplitudes were likewise derived in a peak-to-peak fashion. The values represent means and standard errors of 12 subjects (250 ms condition) and 10 subjects (100 ms condition)

| Spatial frequency | 8 c/deg | | 2 c/deg | |
|---|---|---|---|---|
| Drug \ Duration | 250 ms | 100 ms | 250 ms | 100 ms |
| Flurazepam | 0.81 ± 0.04 | 0.91 ± 0.04 | 0.85 ± 0.06 | 0.93 ± 0.05 |
| Lormetazepam | 1.02 ± 0.08 | 1.05 ± 0.07 | 0.98 ± 0.05 | 1.03 ± 0.04 |

VEPs. The VEPs elicited by the two types of gratings (2 and 8 c/deg) can thus serve as indicators of drug action on the movement- and pattern-specific subsystems.

Flurazepam appears to reduce the amplitudes of all VEP components, but lormetazepam had no significant effect on the VEP components when compared to placebo. The action of flurazepam is also specific to the spatial frequency of the gratings, in that it reduced the VEP response to 8 c/deg more than to 2 c/deg. Even though this observation may point to the selectivity of the flurazepam action for the pattern-specific subsystem, the amplitude reduction may also reflect some indirect effect of flurazepam. In order to exclude the possibility that flurazepam reduced the amplitudes to 8 c/deg gratings by interfering with the accuracy ot the subject's accommodation, we made an additional set of measurements with gratings presented for 100 ms. Brief presentations, however, produce a superposition of the on- and off-set related VEP components and thus generate a complex wave containing both pattern- and movement-related components (see Kulikowski 1972). Table 2 shows that decreasing the stimulus exposure from 250 to 100 ms reduced the size of the attenuation effect of flurazepam on the VEP amplitudes generated by 8 c/deg gratings.

## 4 Discussion

Results presented here allow us to conclude that both the visual and late EP components seem to provide a sensitive indicator of benzodiazepine action on the CNS. The interpretation of such effects is, however, difficult principally due to the patchy state of the present knowledge concerning the mechanism of drug action on the neural structures generating measurable EP components and localization of the origins of the various cognitive or merely the visual EP components. The VEPs elicited by gratings probably originate in the occipital region of the brain encompassing striate and extrastriate areas of the visual cortex. Their origins can, however, only be indirectly inferred from the locations and orientations of current dipoles determined by measuring visual evoked neuromagnetic fields to gratings (Blum et al. 1983). In our study, repeated flurazepam ingestion reduced the responses of both the pattern- and movement-related components which suggests nonspecificity of the drug action.

The origin of the late components contingent on performing a discrimination task are as yet uncertain. Some investigators have even suggested that P300 may originate from the hippocampus (Okada et al. 1983). Yet the acceptance of the supposed origin of the P300 component in the hippocampus needs additional qualification concerning the type of the P300 or N200 one records; unless we, of course, make the unlikely assumption that N200 and P300 components generated in various tasks and recorded from a number of different locations are all the same. This seems, however, improbable since two different N200 waves (one related to the reaction time, the other one not) were recorded from two separate locations, CZ and POZ (Renault et al. 1982). Our results may also indicate that a discrimination task produces at least two types of N200 and two types of P300 waves with different sensitivities to the action of flurazepam. The sources of these waves in the parieto-occipital region must be separate since the N200 and P300 amplitudes are less attenuated in the occipital than in the parietal recording sites. Note, that the occipital P300 is attenuated to a similar degree as the VEP elicited by fine gratings (8 c/deg).

The hangover effect of flurazepam on both visual and cognitive EP components indicates a high degree of nonspecificity. Flurazepam seems to attenuate both the pattern and movement responses of the visual system and also to affect cognitive functions, reaction times and sensitivity to flicker (see also Ciesielski et al. 1983). This broad range of flurazepam action is not surprising since benzodiazepine receptors are distributed all over the human brain (Young and Kuhar 1979). Even though its action seems nonspecific as far as the distribution of the binding sites in the brain is concerned, because of the differences in the attenua-

**Table 3.** Relative effects of flurazepam on various parameters 12 h after the last oral administration. The relative effect (%) is defined here as a coefficient of (flurazepam-placebo)/placebo. The N-desalkylflurazepam effect on EP amplitudes to amoeboid figures and gratings, and the effect on RTs during the discrimination task where the priority was accuracy rather than speed were measured in the present study. Other tabulated values (*), obtained under similar conditions (Ciesielski et al. 1983) were included for the sake of comparison

| Evoked potentials (EP) | | | | | | | |
|---|---|---|---|---|---|---|---|
| Amoeboid shapes | | | | | Gratings (8 c/deg) | | |
| Sites | Parietal | | Occipital | | Occipital | | |
| Waves | P300 | N200 | P300 | N200 | Duration | 250 ms | 100 ms |
| | − 31% | − 26% | − 19% | − 18% | | − 19% | − 9% |
| Reaction times | | | | | | | |
| Discrimination task | | | | | Flash detection task* | | |
| Priority | Speed* | | Accuracy | | Speed | | |
| | + 12% | | + 5% | | + 10% | | |
| Response to flicker | | | | | | | |
| Flicker sensitivity* | | | | | CFF* | | |
| − 7% | | | | | − 3% | | |

tion of the various sensory and cognitive functions, the affinity of flurazepam for the underlying neural subsystems cannot be the same (see Table 3) and may, in part, be attributed to the heterogeneity of benzodiazepine binding sites (Williams et al. 1980; Squires 1981). For instance, neural structures underlying flicker detection are the least susceptible to the action of flurazepam, whereas structure responsible for the amplitude of the parietal P300 wave is the most sensitive (see also Kranda 1982; Ciesielski et al. 1983). Table 3 shows that the spectrum of the effect magnitude of flurazepam is almost continuous.

Because of its short half-life, lormetazepam does not accumulate in the body and thus, even after five consecutive doses, we were unable to detect any appreciable effect 12 h after the last oral administration. If anything, lormetazepam may induce a slight rebound effect (see Table 2). Since the major active metabolite of flurazepam, N-desalkylflurazepam, has an average half-life of about 70 h (range 47–100 h) repeated doses of flurazepam lead to the accumulation of this metabolite. The concentration of N-desalkylflurazepam after five days becomes equivalent to about three times of the original 30 mg flurazepam dose. We were surprised that chronic administration of flurazepam was, after five doses, less effective in suppressing the amplitudes of the N200 and P300 waves than a single dose (see Ciesielski et al. 1983 for comparative values). The diminishing return from flurazepam may reflect some kind of adaptation process in the neural structures whose functions we have measured here, but it may also result from the slightly different (possibly causing less stress to the subject) discrimination task used in the present study (cf. Pfefferbaum et al. 1983 for a comparison of P300 amplitudes).

The observed flurazepam and N-desalkylflurazepam effects on the amplitudes of the VEPs are probably in some way related to the reduction in the stimulus detectability. Flurazepam and N-desalkylflurazepam probably directly inhibit some neurons in structures processing and/or detecting the presented stimuli by acting on the chloride ion channel (Costa et al. 1979) and in this way may reduce the magnitude of neural responses. An amplitude reduction may also reflect a desynchronization of two or more components in a single EP wave. The size of the P300 amplitudes is supposed to be inversely proportional to the subjective probability of the stimuli (see Donchin et al. 1978 for a review of this argument) and directly related to the complexity of the decision task (Picton et al. 1978). The amplitudes of N200 and P300 waves are also proportional to the value of the bet (U.S.-$) in a computerized gambling task (Sutton 1979) and presumably related to the state of excitation or perhaps anxiety. Since a number of factors seem to determine the amplitude sizes of the late EP waves, we cannot at present offer an elegant interpretation of the flurazepam effect on these components. The observed amplitude attenuation may either represent an impairment of the discrimination performance or reflect a sedating effect of flurazepam which damps the excitement or anxiety associated with the experiment. If the observed amplitude reduction were simply a product of flurazepam's anxiolytic properties, then benzodiazepine antagonists such as Ro 15-1788 and FG 7142 (Hunkeler et al. 1981; Dorow et al. 1983) should have an opposite effect. A rebound effect observed after administration of very short-acting benzodiazepines should likewise increase the level of excitement and thus the amplitudes of the late EP components.

## References

Besser GM (1967) Time course of action of diazepam. Nature 214:428
Blum T, Bauer R, Bente D (1983) Investigations of the retinotopic organization of the human visual cortex using the neuromagnetic method. In: Nodar RH, Barber C (eds) Evoked potentials II. Butterworth, New York
Ciesielski KT (1982) Lateralization of visual cognitive potentials. Biol Psychol 14:259–270
Ciesielski KT, Kulikowski JJ, Kranda K, Alvarez SL, Ott H (1983) The hangover effects of benzodiazepines on cognitive and visual functions. In: Benzodiazepines, sleep and daytime performance. Medicine Publishing Foundation, Oxford
Costa T, Rodbard D, Pert CB (1979) Is the benzodiazepine receptor coupled to a chloride anion channel? Nature 277:315–317
Donchin E, Ritter W, McCallum C (1978) Cognitive psychophysiology: the endogenous components of the ERP. In: Callaway E, Tueting P, Koslow S (eds) Brain event-related potentials in man. Academic Press, New York, pp 349–441
Dorow RG, Seidler J, Schneider HH (1982) A radioreceptor assay to study the affinity of benzodiazepines and their binding activity in human plasma including their active metabolites. Br J Clin Pharmacol 13:561–565
Dorow RG, Horowski R, Paschelke G, Amin M, Braestrup C (1983) Severe anxiety induced by FG 7142, a $\beta$-carboline ligand for benzodiazepine receptors. Lancet 8341:98–99
Greenblatt DJ, Shader RI, Divoll M, Harmatz JS (1981) Benzodiazepines: a summary of pharmacokinetic properties. Br J Clin Pharmacol 11:11–16
Hunkeler W, Möhler H, Pieri L, Polc P, Bonetti EP, Schaffner R, Haefely W (1981) Selective antagonists of benzodiazepines. Nature 290:514–516
Kaplan SA, Jack ML (1983) Metabolism of the benzodiazepines: Pharmacokinetic and pharmacodynamic considerations. In: Costa E (ed) The benzodiazepines: from molecular biology to clinical practice. Raven Press, New York, pp 173–199
Kranda K (1982) Potential applications of various flicker techniques in psychopharmacology: The aims and limits. In: Ott H, Kranda K (eds) Flicker techniques in psychopharmacology. Beltz Verlag, Weinheim Basel, pp 14–22
Kulikowski JJ (1972) Relation of psychophysics and electrophysiology. Trace (Paris) 6:64–69
Kulikowski JJ (1976) Methods for separating pattern- and movement-related evoked potentials. J Physiol (Lond) 257:35–36
Kulikowski JJ (1978a) Pattern and movement detection in man and rabbit: separation and comparison of occipital potentials. Vision Res 18:183–189
Kulikowski JJ (1978b) Spatial resolution for the detection of pattern and movement (real and apparent) Vision Res 18:237–238
Kulikowski JJ, Leisman G (1973) The effect of nitrous oxide on the relation between the evoked potential and contrast threshold. Vision Res 13:2079–2086
Okada YC, Kaufman L, Williamson SJ (1983) The hippocampal formation as a source of the slow endogenous potentials. Electroencephalogr Clin Neurophysiol 55:417–426
Pfefferbaum A, Ford J, Johnson R, Wenegrat B, Kopell BS (1983) Manipulation of P3 latency: speed vs. accuracy instructions. Electroencephalogr Clin Neurophysiol 55:188–197
Picton IW, Campbell KB, Baribeau-Braun J, Proulx GB (1978) The neurophysiology of human attention: a tutorial review. In: Requin J (ed) Attention and performance, VII. Erlbaum, Hillsdale, N J, pp 429–467
Renault B, Ragot R, Lesevre N, Remond A (1982) Onset and offset of brain events as indices of mental chronometry. Science 215:1413–1415
Squires RF (1981) GABA receptors regulate the affinities of anions required for brain specific benzodiazepine binding. Adv Biochem Psychopharmacol 26:129–138
Sutton S (1979) P300 - Thirteen years later. In: Begleiter H (ed) Evoked brain potentials and behaviour. Plenum Press, New York London
Williams EF, Rice KC, Paul SM, Skolnick P (1980) Heterogeneity of benzodiazepine receptors in the central nervous system demonstrated with kenazepine, an alkylating benzodiazepine. J Neurochem 35:591–597
Young WS III, Kuhar MJ (1979) Autoradiographic localization of benzodiazepine receptors in the brains of humans and animals. Nature 280:393–395

# Amnesic Effects of Lormetazepam

T. Roehrs, A. McLenaghan, G. Koshorek, F. Zorick and T. Roth[1]

**Contents**



**Abstract**

Sixteen healthy men, age 18–35, each received lormetazepam (1.5 mg), flurazepam (30 mg), temazepam (30 mg) and placebo (double-blind in a Latin Square design) 30 min before bedtime for 2 consecutive nights followed by a 12 day washout between conditions. Three hours after drug (2.5 h after bedtime) subjects were awakened and administered a 16-item memory task. Fifteen minutes after the awakening subjects returned to bed, were instructed to go to sleep, and remained in bed for an additional 5.5 h. Immediately after the memory tasks, before returning to bed, subjects recalled almost all of the 16 items when placebo was administered before bedtime. Immediate recall was significantly poorer than placebo after temazepam and flurazepam, but not after lormetazepam. Morning recall was reduced significantly from the immediate nighttime level in each condition; this loss was smallest with placebo. All active drug conditions produced significantly greater amnesia than placebo. This amnesia was smallest after lormetazepam and greatest after temazepam, which differed significantly from each other. All active drugs significantly reduced latency measures of the return to sleep after the 15 min awakening; it was shortest with temazepam and longest with flurazepam. This study showed a relation between the hypnotic and amnesic effects of these drugs which is consistent with their pharmacokinetic properties.

**Key Words**

Anterograde amnesia/Daytime residual effects/Disruption of performance tasks/EEG/EMG/EOG/Flurazepam/Immediate recall/Memory test/Morning recall/REM sleep/Safety parameters/Sleep latency/Temazepam.

---

1 Sleep Disorders and Research Center, Henry Ford Hospital, Detroit, MI 48202, USA

Psychopharmacology Supplementum 1
Editors: I. Hindmarch, H. Ott and T. Roth

# 1 Introduction

Lormetazepam, the N-methyl derivative of lorazepam, has hypnotic properties as demonstrated using polysomnographic methods in healthy young adults and in patients with insomnia (Nicholson and Stone 1982; Oswald et al. 1979). Over the dose range 0.5, 1.0, 2.0 and 2.5 mg lormetazepam increased total sleep time and reduced wakefulness and drowsy sleep (stage 1). But in clinical use, sedative activity must be balanced against other undesired effects associated with these compounds.

One important safety consideration in the use of these compounds is the extent to which they produce amnesic effects. There is evidence that some benzodiazepines produce anterograde amnesia, amnesia for events occuring subsequent to administration of the drug. Three recent studies of amnesia following benzodiazepine hypnotic use found disturbed morning recall for tasks presented during a nighttime awakening three hours after administration of the drug (Roth et al. 1980; Bixler et al. 1979; Roehrs et al. in press). Among those benzodiazepines producing amnesia was lorazepam, the precursor of lormetazepam.

Another safety consideration involves the degree of continued pharmacologic activity during the day following nighttime administration. These residual effects are related primarily to the half-life of the parent compound or its active metabolites, but dosage also can affect duration of activity. While the half-life of lormetazepam is 10–15 h (Hümpel et al. 1979), one study has reported residual effects following 2.0 mg (Nicholson and Stone 1982) and another study found no residual effects the next day with 2.5 mg (Oswald et al. 1979). Since hypnotic effects are present with low doses (0.5 and 1.0 mg), but residual effects may occur with higher doses, a 1.5 mg dose may be the optimally effective and safe dose.

This study evaluated the amnesic properties and daytime residual effects of lormetazepam (1.5 mg) in comparison to flurazepam (30 mg) and temazepam (30 mg). Of secondary interest were the sleep induction and sleep maintenance properties of lormetazepam in comparison to flurazepam and temazepam.

# 2 Methods

## 2.1 Subjects

Sixteen healthy men, age 18–35, volunteered for the study and signed an informed consent. All were in good health based on the results of a physical examination, history and clinical laboratory tests. Candidates were excluded if there was evidence of significant gastrointestinal, hepatic, renal, or other system abnormalities, or a history of drug addiction, alcoholism, known hypersensitivity to benzodiazepines, or if they required concomitant CNS medication during the study.

## 2.2 Design

Lormetazepam (1.5 mg), flurazepam (30 mg), temazepam (30 mg) and placebo were administered, double-blind, according to a Latin Square design. The subjects received each experimental condition on each of two nights with a twelve day washout between conditions.

### 2.3 Procedure

On each experimental night, subjects reported to the laboratory at least one hour before their usual sleep time. Electrodes were attached for continuous monitoring of the central and occipital EEGs, electrooculogram (EOG), and the submental electromyogram (EMG). Thirty minutes prior to lights out and the initiation of the all-night recording, subjects took their medication.

Three hours after administration of the capsules (2.5 h after lights out), each subject was awakened by calling his name over the intercom. The wake-up call was repeated until at least 30 s of polysomnographic signs of wake were observed. The technician immediately entered the room, turned on the lights, and questioned the subject to verify that he was awake. Then the subject was seated at a desk for the presentation of the memory test.

The memory test consisted of a series of four tasks, each containing four details. This memory test, its rationale, its split-half reliability, and its test-retest reliability have been described previously (Roth et al. 1980). Briefly, the tasks were

1) a pill task in which subjects ingested small mints (different than the real medication) and recalled the color of the mint container, the number and color of the mints;
2) a dressing task in which subjects put articles of clothing on and recalled the names of two articles, the color of one, and the sequence of dressing;
3) a travel task in which details of a hypothetical journey including destination, name of airline, time of departure, and flight number were to be remembered; and
4) a clock task requiring memory for the pre-set time on a clock, the color of the clock, the type of numerals on the clock face, and the time to which the subject reset the clock.

The relevant details of each task were changed nightly to preclude any improvement in memory over nights. A five digit number also was presented during each awakening following the memory test.

After completing all tasks, each subject completed a 17-item questionnaire which assessed his memory for the four details of the four tasks and the five digit number. Fifteen minutes after the awakening, subjects returned to bed, lights were turned out and the recording was resumed. Subjects were instructed to go to sleep and remained in bed for an additional 5.5 h (a total recording of 8 h).

In the morning on arising, memory for the 17-item memory test was assessed. At this time subjects also completed a post-sleep questionnaire. After dressing and a small breakfast (decaffeinated coffee and a muffin) subjects took a performance battery. The battery included simple reaction time, complex reaction time, memory span, divided attention, digit symbol substitution, digit symbol copying, and vigilance tasks.

All patients were instructed not to consume alcohol or any other medication during the course of the study. On all nights coffee, tea or cola were not allowed after 7.30 p.m. Also, naps were not permitted during the study.

The mean of the two nights of each experimental condition for each subject was computed for all safety parameters (middle-of-night memory and next morning performance). Each polysomnographic recording was scored manually in 30 s epochs according to the standards of Rechtschaffen and Kales (1968), and means were computed for all sleep parameters. To compare the four experimental conditions on each safety and sleep parameter, ANOVAs (repeated measures) were conducted and post hoc comparisons were made using the Duncan's multiple range test.

## 3 Results

### 3.1 Safety Parameters

The anterograde amnesic effects of lormetazepam compared to temazepam and flurazepam are summarized in Table 1.

Immediately after the memory tasks, subjects recalled almost all of the 16 items when placebo was administered before bedtime. Immediate recall was significantly poorer than placebo with temazepam and flurazepam, but not with lormetazepam. Morning recall was reduced significantly from the immediate nighttime level in each condition; this loss from night to morning was smallest with placebo. All active drug conditions produced significantly greater amnesia than placebo. This amnesia was smallest after lormetazepam and greatest after temazepam; the difference between lormetazepam and temazepam was significant. These differential drug effects on amnesia are illustrated in Fig. 1. Results for recall of the 5-digit number were in the same direction as those of the 16-item memory task, but these differences were not statistically significant.

Table 2 summarizes the data on the morning residual effects of lormetazepam compared to temazepam and flurazepam. Performance of complex tasks (complex RT, central RT and peripheral RT in the divided attention task, and DSST) was disrupted significantly following nighttime administration of flurazepam. In contrast, after temazepam, except for DSST which was reduced significantly,

**Table 1.** Middle-of-night memory

| | Placebo | Lormetazepam (1.5 mg) | Temazepam (30 mg) | Flurazepam (30 mg) |
|---|---|---|---|---|
| Number recalled night | 15.1 ± 1.41 | 14.4 ± 1.15 | 13.8 ± 2.22[a] | 14.2 ± 1.75[a] |
| Number recalled morning | 14.6 ± 1.20[c] | 12.6 ± 1.85[a,c] | 11.2 ± 3.39[a,b,c] | 11.8 ± 2.96[a,c] |
| Digits recalled night | 4.5 ± 0.77 | 4.6 ± 0.74 | 3.9 ± 1.39 | 3.9 ± 1.31 |
| Digits recalled morning | 4.1 ± 1.19 | 3.8 ± 1.15 | 3.5 ± 1.66 | 3.5 ± 1.47 |

[a] Differs from placebo, $p < 0.05$ Duncan's post hoc range test
[b] Differs from lormetazepam, $p < 0.05$ Duncan's post hoc range test
[c] Differs from night, t test $p < 0.05$

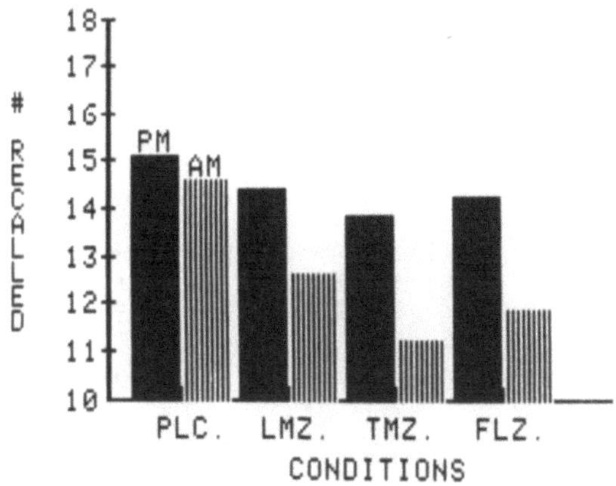


**Fig. 1.** Number of items recalled for each drug condition in the middle of the night and in the morning

**Table 2.** Next morning performance

| | Placebo | Lormetazepam (1.5 mg) | Temazepam (30 mg) | Flurazepam (30 mg) |
|---|---|---|---|---|
| Simple RT | 452 ± 126 | 459 ± 115 | 504 ± 203 | 482 ± 115 |
| Complex RT | 650 ± 109 | 653 ± 120 | 646 ± 102 | 692 ± 120[a–c] |
| Memory span | | | | |
| Corr 8 digits | 6.6 ± 1.5 | 6.7 ± 1.2 | 6.3 ± 1.7 | 6.4 ± 1.7 |
| Corr 9 digits | 6.7 ± 1.8 | 6.6 ± 1.8 | 6.4 ± 2.0 | 6.2 ± 2.0 |
| Total corr | 24.6 ± 5.7 | 24.9 ± 5.0 | 24.2 ± 5.5 | 24.1 ± 5.6 |
| Divided Attention | | | | |
| Av track | 115 ± 41 | 112 ± 35 | 99 ± 19 | 111 ± 40 |
| SS track | 2192 | 2100 | 1888 | 2327 |
| Central RT | 26.8 ± 4.7 | 27.2 ± 4.9 | 26.9 ± 4.3 | 30.0 ± 8.4[a–c] |
| Peripheral RT | 25.9 ± 4.9 | 26.2 ± 5.3 | 25.7 ± 4.1 | 30.3 ± 8.5[a–c] |
| DSST (corr) | 176.1 ± 37.5 | 177.3 ± 43.4 | 165.5 ± 37.0[a,b] | 151.3 ± 37.4[a–c] |
| DSCT (corr) | 359.3 ± 79.3 | 370.1 ± 88.9 | 358.3 ± 72.1 | 368.1 ± 83.9 |
| Vigilance | | | | |
| RT quart 1 | 783 ± 316 | 837 ± 391 | 707 ± 356 | 727 ± 310 |
| RT quart 2 | 869 ± 303 | 841 ± 435 | 878 ± 355 | 810 ± 355 |
| RT quart 3 | 874 ± 326 | 861 ± 368 | 860 ± 396 | 951 ± 429 |
| RT quart 4 | 865 ± 317 | 877 ± 355 | 863 ± 360 | 909 ± 409 |
| Total errors | 5.3 ± 6.4 | 7.2 ± 7.3 | 5.6 ± 7.6 | 11.9 ± 12.2[a–c] |

[a] Differs from placebo, $p < 0.05$ Duncan's post hoc range test
[b] Differs from lormetazepam, $p < 0.05$ Duncan's post hoc range test
[c] Differs from temazepam, $p < 0.05$ Duncan's post hoc range test

performance was unaltered. Finally, none of the performance measures were affected by lormetazepam.

### 3.2 Effects on Sleep

The effects of lormetazepam, temazepam and flurazepam on sleep are presented in Table 3. While the subjects were healthy individuals without sleeping problems

**Table 3.** Polysomnographic measures

| | Placebo | Lormetazepam (1.5 mg) | Temazepam (30 mg) | Flurazepam (30 mg) |
|---|---|---|---|---|
| *Hypnotic effects* | | | | |
| 1) Initial induction | | | | |
| Lat to 2 | 19.5 ± 15.6 | 15.6 ± 7.2 | 13.5 ± 5.3 | 20.2 ± 8.4 |
| Lat to Pers Sl | 18.7 ± 13.9 | 12.9 ± 6.1 | 10.9 ± 6.2 | 17.0 ± 10.0 |
| WBS | 15.0 ± 13.5 | 10.8 ± 5.7 | 9.0 ± 5.2 | 15.0 ± 8.9 |
| 2) Return induction | | | | |
| Lat to 1 | 8.6 ± 7.0 | 4.9 ± 4.3[a] | 4.1 ± 7.2[a] | 5.5 ± 6.2[a] |
| Lat to 2 | 15.0 ± 11.7 | 9.2 ± 5.7[a] | 8.6 ± 7.3[a] | 9.7 ± 8.2[a] |
| Lat to Pers Sl | 10.9 ± 7.0 | 6.7 ± 5.4[a] | 6.0 ± 7.6[a] | 6.8 ± 6.0[a] |
| 3) Maintenance | | | | |
| WDS | 22.4 ± 19.1 | 12.5 ± 11.0[a] | 17.0 ± 11.1 | 12.5 ± 13.5[a] |
| WAS | 1.5 ± 4.3 | 1.4 ± 2.9 | 2.2 ± 7.0 | 0.5 ± 1.5 |
| # Awak | 4.1 ± 3.0 | 3.1 ± 2.3 | 4.0 ± 2.5 | 3.8 ± 3.4 |
| 4) Overall | | | | |
| TST | 442 ± 29.5 | 455 ± 13.5 | 452 ± 17.5 | 452 ± 20.4 |
| % W | 8.1 ± 6.2 | 5.1 ± 2.8 | 5.9 ± 3.7 | 5.8 ± 4.3 |
| *Sleep staging effects* | | | | |
| % 1 | 11.7 ± 8.1 | 9.3 ± 5.4[a] | 10.0 ± 6.2 | 8.5 ± 5.2[a] |
| % 2 | 56.3 ± 8.0 | 61.3 ± 7.3[a] | 62.5 ± 6.6[a] | 62.4 ± 7.8[a] |
| % 3–4 | 12.6 ± 7.7 | 10.8 ± 7.1 | 10.0 ± 6.9 | 11.1 ± 7.8 |
| % REM | 19.3 ± 5.5 | 18.5 ± 3.6 | 17.4 ± 3.2 | 17.9 ± 4.0 |
| Lat REM | 103 ± 33.5 | 110 ± 28.2 | 156 ± 50.0[a,b] | 137 ± 56.4[a,b] |

[a] Differs from placebo, $p < 0.05$ Duncan's post hoc range test
[b] Differs from lormetazepam, $p < 0.05$ Duncan's post hoc range test

and their sleep was disrupted artificially for the primary purposes of this study, an indication of lormetazepam's comparative hypnotic effects can be obtained from these data.

Initial sleep induction parameters were not reduced significantly from placebo levels with any of the active drugs. However, all active drugs significantly reduced latency measures of the return to sleep after the 15 min awakening (Fig. 2). These latencies were shortest with temazepam and longest with flurazepam. The only measure of sleep maintenance affected by the drugs was wake time during sleep (WDS). WDS was reduced significantly by lormetazepam and flurazepam. None of the active drugs had a significant effect on total sleep time or percent wake time for the 8 h recording.

Benzodiazepines have been shown to affect sleep staging in both healthy normals and patients. In the present study, there was a significant reduction of percent stage 1 sleep with lormetazepam and flurazepam. Percent stage 2 sleep was increased by all three active drugs. The latency to REM sleep increased significantly with temazepam and flurazepam as opposed to both placebo and lormetazepam.

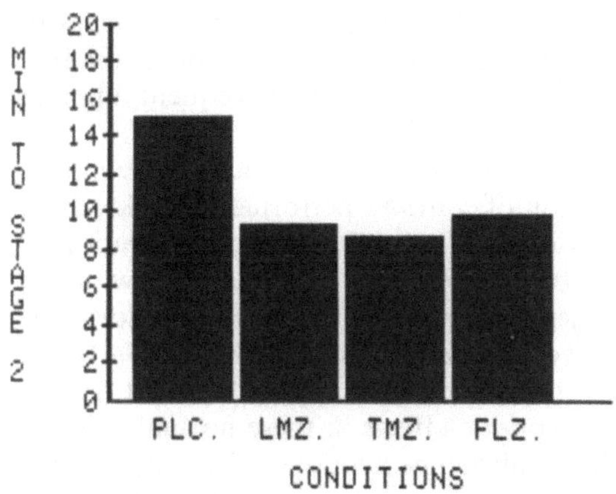


**Fig. 2.** Latency to return to sleep (latency to stage 2 sleep) in each drug condition

### 3.3 Relation of Sleep Induction and Amnesia

We have hypothesized that the mechanism producing amnesia is a failure of memory consolidation at night due to rapid sleep onset following the nighttime awakening. Thus, one would expect that differences in pharmacokinetics and dose equivalency may produce small differences in sleep latency and amnesic effects. There were small differences among drugs in sleep onset after the awakening (see Fig. 2). These differences corresponded with their amnesic effects. The relation between sleep latency after the nighttime awakening and recall of the memory task in the morning is illustrated in Fig. 3. The correlation between sleep latency and morning recall was 0.86 ($p < 0.001$).

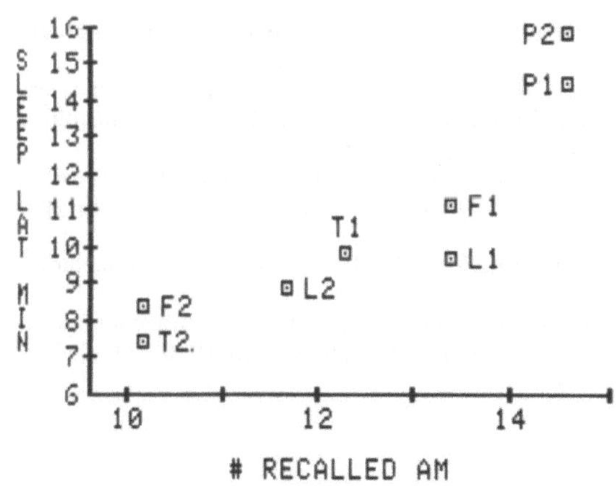


**Fig. 3.** Relation of sleep latency and number of items recalled in the morning

## 4 Discussion

Lormetazepam compared favorably in its safety characteristics with the other two benzodiazepine hypnotics. It produces anterograde amnesia as the others, but its amnesic effect was the smallest among the active drugs. However, the point must be made that these differences may reflect small differences among the drugs in pharmacokinetics and dose equivalency. At one hour or four hours post administration, a somewhat different pattern of sleep latencies and consequent amnesic effects may have been seen.

In the morning no residual effects of lormetazepam were found. In contrast flurazepam produced significant disruption of complex performance tasks. Such residual effects have been reported previously after nighttime administration of flurazepam (Bond and Lader 1973). These differences are consistent with the known pharmacokinetics of these two benzodiazepines. The half-life of lormetazepam is 10–15 h and flurazepam's active metabolite has a half-life of 47–100 h.

Lormetazepam's safety at the 1.5 mg dose does not appear to result from a sacrifice in its hypnotic properties. Its hypnotic effects in these normal subjects were similar to those of the other two benzodiazepine hypnotics. As well, its effect on sleep stages was quite similar to the effects of flurazepam and temazepam. The one noteable exception was latency to REM sleep which increased with both temazepam and flurazepam, but was not changed with lormetazepam. This again may reflect small differences in pharmacokinetics.

## References

Bixler EO, Scharf MB, Soldatos CR, Mitsky DJ, Kales A (1979) Effects of hypnotic drugs on memory. Life Sci 25:1379–1388

Bond AJ, Lader MH (1973) Residual effects of flurazepam. Psychopharmacologia 32:223–235

Hümpel M, Illi V, Milius W, Wendt H, Kurowski M (1979) The pharmacokinetics and biotransformation of the new benzodiazepine lormetazepam in humans. 1. Absorption, distribution, elimination and metabolism of lormetazepam-5-$^{14}C$. Eur J Drug Metab Pharmacokinet 4:237–243

Nicholson AN, Stone BM (1982) Hypnotic activity and effects on performance of lormetazepam and camazepam – analogues of temazepam. Br J Clin Pharmocol 13:433–439

Oswald I, Adam K, Borrow S, Idzikowski C (1979) The effects of two hypnotics on sleep, subjective feelings and skilled performance. In: Passouant P, Oswald I (eds) Pharmacology of the states of alertness. Pergamon Press, Oxford, pp 51–63

Rechtschaffen A, Kales A (1968) A manual of standardized terminology, techniques and scoring system for sleep stages of human subjects. National Institute of Health Publication, No. 204. U.S. Government Printing Office, Washington, DC

Roehrs T, Zorick F, Sicklesteel J, Wittig R, Hartse K, Roth T. Effects of hypnotics on memory. J Clin Psychopharm (in press)

Roth T, Hartse KM, Saab PG, Piccione PM, Kramer M (1980) The effects of flurazepam, lorazepam and triazolam on sleep and memory. Psychopharmacology (Berlin) 70:231–237

# The Effects of Benzodiazepines on Short-Term Memory and Information Processing

Z. Subhan [1]

**Contents**



**Abstract**

The effects of flunitrazepam 1 mg, triazolam 0.25 mg, lormetazepam 1 mg and placebo on stages of information processing in a Sternberg memory scanning task were investigated in ten normal volunteers.

Overall reaction times for the task were increased 1 h following treatment with triazolam and both 1 h and 10 h following treatment with flunitrazepam. Response latencies were not appreciably altered by lormetazepam or placebo.

The effects of flunitrazepam and triazolam were found to be localised in the stimulus encoding and serial comparison stages of the reaction process and not in response-selection organisation.

**Key Words**

Alcohol/Anterograde amnesia/Dual theory of memory/Flunitrazepam/Hangover/Lormetazepam/Methaqualone/Nitrazepam/Response latencies/Response selection/Secobarbital/Stages of information processing/Sternberg memory scanning task/Stimulus encoding/Temazepam/Triazolam.

## 1 Introduction

In recent years much interest has focused on the impairment of human memory by the benzodiazepine derivatives. Clearly, with respect to the use of these drugs in clinical examination and procedures involving discomfort, the anterograde amnesia often reported (Clarke et al. 1970; Heisterkamp and Cohen 1975; Dundee and George 1976) might well be deemed advantageous. However, such an interference of memory would not be a desirable side-effect for patients who take benzodiazepines orally to assist sleep induction or to allay anxiety. Although

1 Human Psychopharmacology Research Unit, University of Leeds, GB-Leeds, LS2 9JT

Psychopharmacology Supplementum 1
Editors: I. Hindmarch, H. Ott and T. Roth

amnesia is most often reported following the intravenous administration of benzodiazepines, several studies have demonstrated drug related effects following oral doses (Bixler et al. 1979; McKay and Dundee 1980; Siegfried et al. 1981; Subhan 1981). A knowledge of such side-effects on memory would seem to be of particular benefit to the physician prescribing hypnotic or sedative drugs to the elderly patients perhaps already experiencing a deterioration of cognitive abilities with age.

According to the dual theory of memory (Atkinson and Shiffrin 1971) incoming information enters a limited capacity short-term memory (STM) where it can be maintained by rehearsal and successfully transferred to long-term memory (LTM) or lost by displacement. In contrast to the relatively permanent LTM, STM therefore refers to memory for information the retrieval of which is requested after intervals of not more than a few minutes in length and often as short as a few seconds. Memory episodes of about this time order are of great practical importance because there are innumerable real-life situations where people must make delayed use of information received some seconds previously.

Using simple tests such as digit span and telephone number recall, an impairment of STM by the benzodiazepines has been demonstrated following acute oral doses of diazepam (Haffner et al. 1973; Mørland et al. 1974; Subhan 1981), temazepam (Liljequist and Mattila 1979) and clobazam (Subhan 1981) and following nocturnal medication with nitrazepam, flurazepam, triazolam and temazepam (Subhan 1982).

However, successful performance in a memory-span task requires more than storage space to hold the items. When the time comes to recall, the items must be retrieved from storage.

Retrieval from STM has been studied primarily with an experimental procedure called memory scanning, developed by Sternberg (1969). Briefly, the task requires a subject to decide whether a visually presented probe digit is or is not a member of a previously memorised set of digits. The subject is to respond "yes" if the test stimulus matches one of the memory set items, and "no" if it does not. The responses are usually made by pushing one of two buttons. The dependent variable is the subject's reaction time (RT) – the time it takes to respond "yes" or "no" after seeing the test stimulus. Specifically, RT is the time that elapsed between the onset of the test stimulus and the subject's response (see Fig. 1). Sternberg (1969) proposed that the reaction process in such a task occurs in a series of at least three additive stages. Assuming that the subject has the memory set stored in STM, the subject must first perceive and encode the test stimulus (stimulus encoding), then that stimulus is compared to the members of the memory set (memory scanning or serial comparison) and finally a response is made on the basis of those comparisons (response selection organisation). The total time taken by these stages is the RT (Fig. 1).

The separation of these stages has been achieved in previous studies (Sternberg 1969, Rundell et al. 1978; Williams et al. 1981), by using stimulus quality variables to control the duration of the encoding stage, varying the number of elements held in short-term storage to control the duration of the memory scanning stage and employing such factors as response probability and stimulus-response compatibility to control the duration of the output stages.

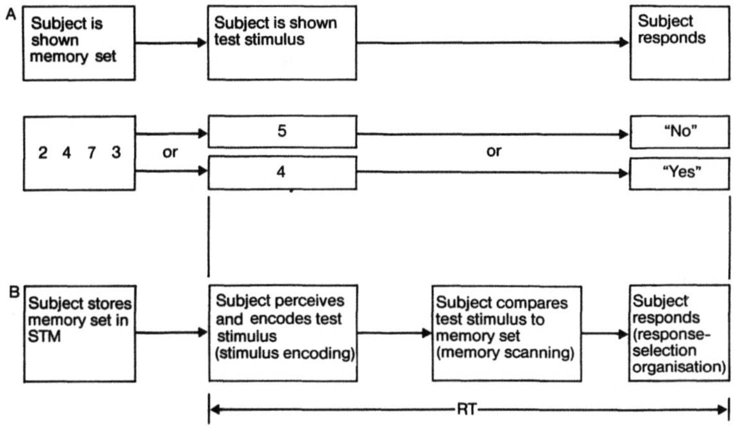


**Fig. 1.** Sternberg's Memory Scanning Task: a) Events of a typical trial, b) proposed mental events during scanning. (From Klatzky, 1980)

Using such a theoretical model of information processing, Rundell et al. (1977, 1978) have established interactions between alcohol and variables defining output processes and secobarbital and methaqualone with variables defining the earlier stimulus-encoding stages of the reaction process. More recently, Williams et al. (1981) examined the effects of secobarbital at two dose levels on reaction times obtained in a memory search task and provided additional evidence for a stage-specific effect of the drug.

The aim of the present study was to examine the acute and residual effects of several benzodiazepine hypnotics on the stages of information processing thought to mediate in a memory scanning task.

## 2 Methods

### 2.1 Subjects

Ten female volunteers aged between 24 and 40 years were admitted to the study. All were in good physical health and without a history of cardiac, renal, hepatic, gastric or mental illness. Actual or possible pregnancy, concurrent medication (excluding the contraceptive pill) or other treatment from a physician precluded participation. Caffeine-containing beverages and alcohol were not permitted for the duration of the study and subjects were not allowed to drive.

### 2.2 Materials

All the medications below were packaged in identical capsules. The four medications were:

- Triazolam 0.25 mg
- Lormetazepam 1 mg
- Flunitrazepam 1 mg
- Placebo.

## 2.3 Design

Each subject acted as her own control and, according to a double-blind crossover design, received one of the four treatments on each study evening. The order of treatment was randomised and balanced with 7 days washout allowed between each test evening.

Individual testing on a memory scanning task (detailed below) took place 1 hour following drug administration after which subjects retired to bed. Further assessment was conducted the following morning (approximately 10 h following treatment administration). Before entry to the trial all subjects received extensive training and familiarisation on the test procedures to preclude learning effects.

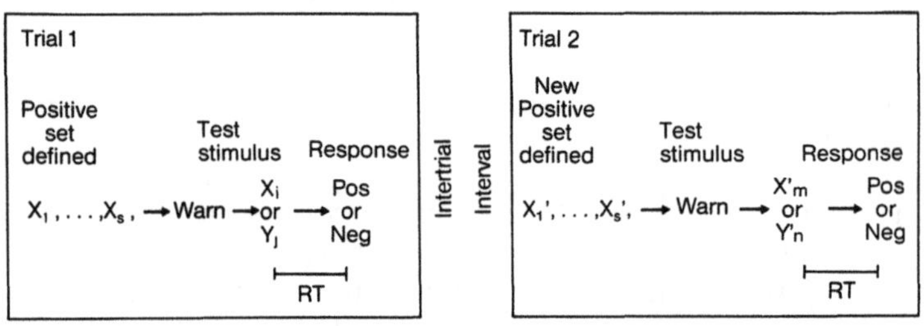


**Fig. 2.** Memory Scanning: Varied-set procedures. A $Y$ represents an item in the negative set. Primes are used in representing trial 2 of the varied-set procedures to show that both the items in the positive set ($X_1, \ldots, X_s$) and its size ($s$) may change from trial to trial. (From Sternberg, 1969)

Figure 2 illustrates the varied set of procedures described by Sternberg (1969) and used in the present study. A microcomputer (Apple II) and video monitor (Hitachi, model VM 906 AE/K) used in conjunction with a BASIC computer programme facilitated presentation of task material, measurement of RT and recording of results.

Subjects were required to memorise series of 4, 5 or 6 digits (positive set) presented sequentially at a 1.2 seconds/digit rate and at two levels of stimulus discriminability. Two seconds after the last digit in the set was displayed, an auditory warning signal (750 ms) duration was sounded followed by a single test (probe) digit. Subjects responded by pressing one of two keys: "yes" (positive response) if the test digit was contained in the memorised list, and "no" (negative response) if it was not. In accordance with the varied-set procedure, a new positive set ranging randomly over trials from 4 to 6 different digits was presented. Each subject was instructed to respond as rapidly as possible without making errors and completed 10 "practice" trials followed by further 48 "experimental" trials. The intertrial interval was 3 s. The two levels of stimulus discriminability were achieved by presenting the probe digit using the normal (high discriminability) and inverse (low discriminability) functions of the microcomputer in random order. Within the 48 trials, there were 36 negative and 12 positive probes. The response measure was the mean correct RT for each treatment for each subject.

## 3 Results

One subject had to withdraw from the study for personal reasons unconnected with the drug treatment. Final analyses were therefore conducted for 9 subjects.

An initial three-way analysis of variance of placebo scores confirmed that there were no significant interaction effects between the variables discriminability (high, low), set size (4, 5 or 6 digits) and response type (positive, negative). Further analyses of the drug effects on overall RT for the memory scanning task revealed significant ($p < 0.05$) increases in response latency 1 h following treatment with flunitrazepam and triazolam and the morning following treatment with flunitrazepam when compared to placebo (Fig. 3).

The effects of the two discriminability conditions 1 h and 10 h following medication are shown in Figs. 4 and 5. There was a significant drug by discriminability interaction at 1 h ($F = 17.8$; $df = 3.24$; $p < 0.0000$) and at 10 h ($F = 16.9$; $df = 3.24$; $p < 0.0000$) post-administration and this was reflected in the highly significant ($p < 0.0000$) simple main effects of discriminability for both flunitrazepam and triazolam of both test times.

Similar results were found for set size (Figs. 8 and 9) and analyses showed significant drug by set size interactions at both 1 h ($F = 12.4$; $df = 6.48$; $p < 0.0000$) and 10 h ($F = 3.0$; $df = 6.48$; $p < 0.01$). Simple main effects of set size for flunitrazepam and triazolam were again highly significant ($p < 0.0000$) both following acute dose and testing the following morning.

Figures 6 and 7 show the joint effects of drug treatment and response type at the two time intervals. In contrast to discriminability and set size, no significant drug response type interactions were found, although at both 1 h and 10 h post-

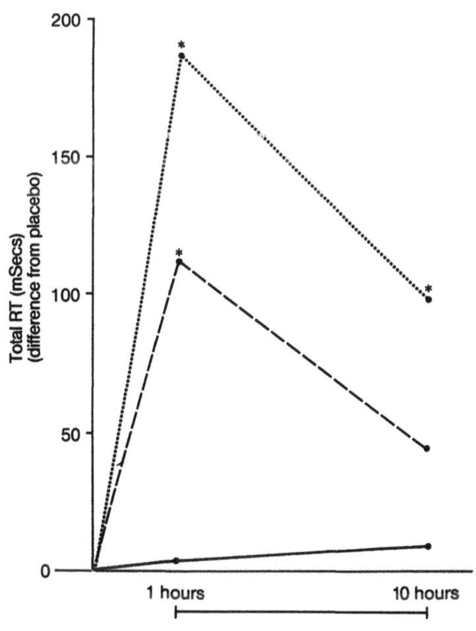


**Fig. 3.** Overall RT (differences from placebo) following treatment with: lormetazepam ●——●, triazolam ● — — ●, flunitrazepam ●-----●, at 1 h and 10 h post-administration ($n = 9$). (* = significant difference from placebo, $p < 0.05$)

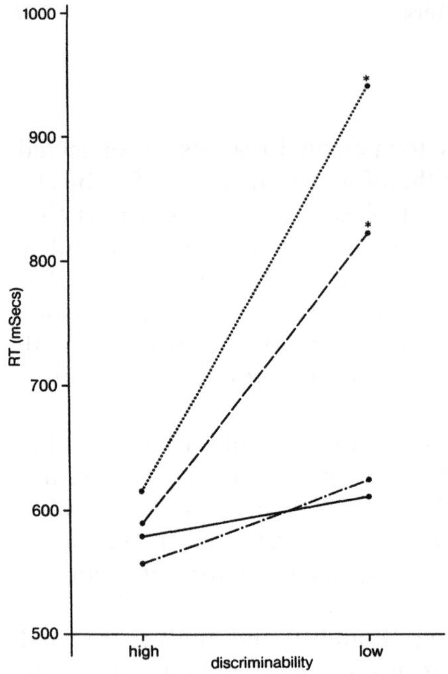


**Fig. 4.** Joint effects of drug and discriminability on RT ($n = 9$) 1 h following treatment with: placebo ●–·–·●, lormetazepam ●——●, triazolam ● – – ●, flunitrazepam ●- - - - -●

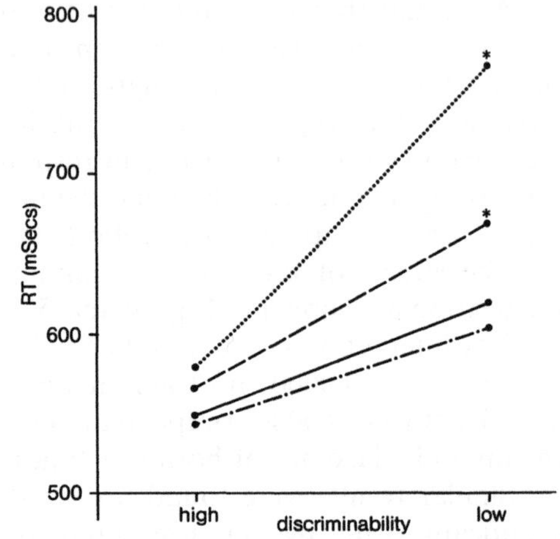


**Fig. 5.** Joint effects of drug and discriminability on RT ($n = 9$) 10 h following treatment with: placebo ●–·–·●, lormetazepam ●——●, triazolam ● – – ●, flunitrazepam ●- - - - -●

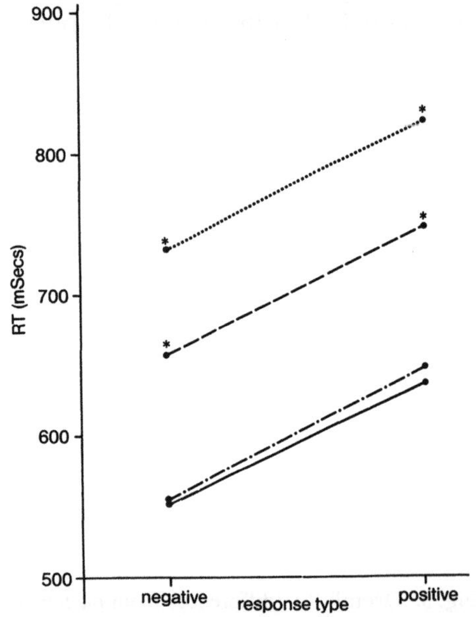


**Fig. 6.** Joint effects of drug and response type on RT ($n = 9$) 1 h following treatment with: placebo ●–·–·●, lormetazepam ●——●, triazolam ● – – ●, flunitrazepam ●- - - - -●

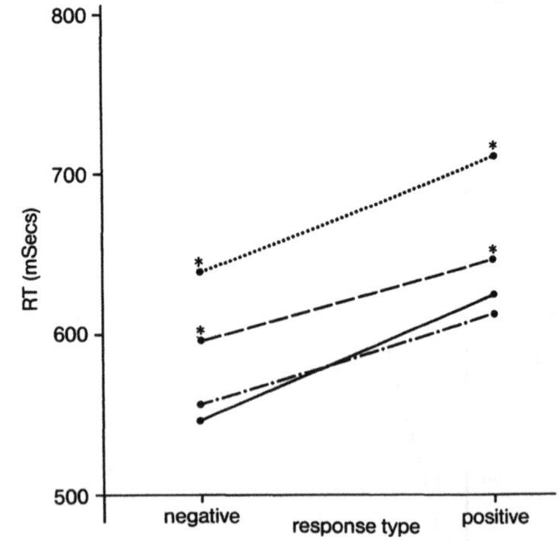


**Fig. 7.** Joint effects of drug and response type on RT ($n = 9$) 10 h following treatment with: placebo ●–·–·●, lormetazepam ●——●, triazolam ● – – ●, flunitrazepam ●- - - - -●

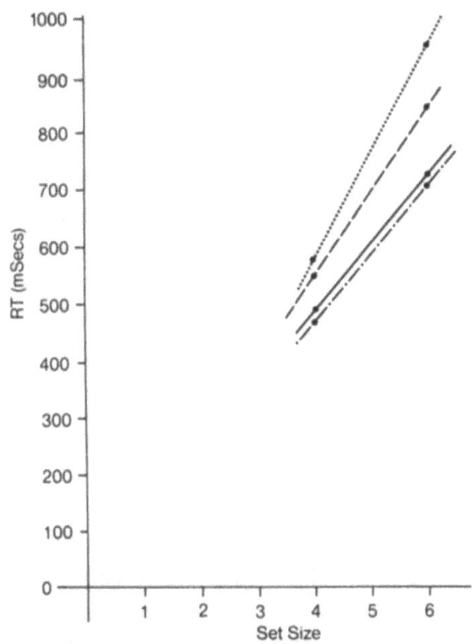


**Fig. 8.** Joint effects of drug and set size on RT ($n = 9$) 1 h following treatment with: placebo ●–·–·●, lormetazepam ●——●, triazolam ● — — ●, flunitrazepam ●-----●

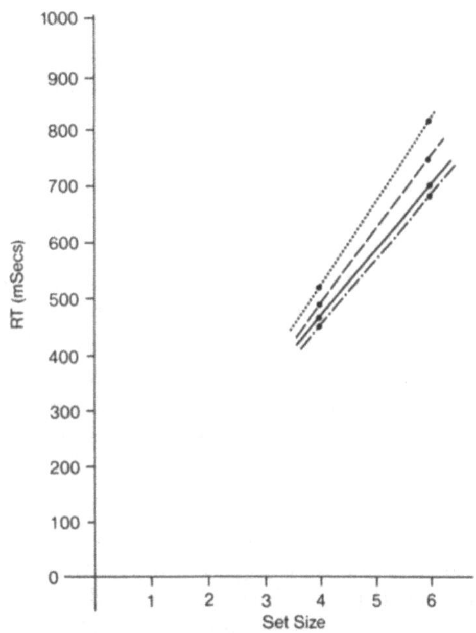


**Fig. 9.** Joint effects of drug and set size on RT ($n = 9$) 10 h following treatment with: placebo ●–·–·●, lormetazepam ●——●, triazolam ● — — ●, flunitrazepam ●-----●

medication, RT's for flunitrazepam and triazolam were significantly longer than placebo for both positive and negative type responses ($p < 0.05$).

## 4 Discussion

The effects of flunitrazepam 1 mg, triazolam 0.25 mg and lormetazepam 1 mg on overall RT for the memory scanning task are clear, with both flunitrazepam and triazolam causing an increase in response latency 1 h following treatment. An increase in overall RT compared to placebo was also noted the morning following medication with flunitrazepam and this is consistent with reports of "hangover" of residual sedative activity following nocturnal medication with benzodiazepines (Bixler et al. 1972; Hindmarch 1976; Roth et al. 1979; Seppälä et al. 1982). No significant changes in overall RT were observed for lormetazepam 1 mg in comparison to placebo and these data are consistent with results from a previous study (Subhan 1982) in which STM capacity (assessed using the digit span test) was unaffected by lormetazepam 1 mg the morning following nighttime ingestion.

The significant drug by discriminability interactions and corresponding highly significant simple main effects for acute doses flunitrazepam and triazolam resulted from increases in RT of 325.5 ms and 234.8 ms respectively in changing from the high to low probe discriminability conditions. Similarly, 10 h following medication, RT's for flunitrazepam increased from 578.3 ms (high discriminability) to 768.2 ms (low discriminability) and triazolam from 567.9 ms to 669.8 ms suggesting drug effects on the first (stimulus encoding) stage of information processing proposed by Sternberg (1969).

As Williams et al. (1981) have pointed out, this encoding stage may also encompass additional activities such as stimulus registration, and it is interesting to note a parallel with previous work (Subhan 1982) suggesting a benzodiazepine-induced decrease in the capacity of the so-called iconic (Sperling 1960) or sensory memory (thought to be implicated in early stimulus registration). The effects of flunitrazepam and triazolam were not, however, isolated in the stimulus encoding stage and are mirrored (although to a lesser extent) in the analysis of RT's for the second, memory scanning or serial comparison stage in which the probe stimulus was compared to each of the members of the memory set. The effect of set size on placebo RT reflected an increase of 116.9 ms in average RT for each digit added to the memory set at 1 h post-medication and 117 ms at 10 h.

In contrast, medication with flunitrazepam resulted in a corresponding increase in RT of 199.8 ms after 1 h and 145 ms the following morning. Similarly for triazolam response latency was increased by 152.4 ms (1 h) and 135.5 ms (10 h). RT's for lormetazepam differed little from placebo.

Reaction times were found to be increased for the less frequent positive probes for all treatment conditions (including placebo), however, in contrast to discriminability and set size variables, there was no evidence to suggest a specific drug effect on the response-selection organisation stage, the separation of which was achieved by the manipulation of response type.

In conclusion, when compared to placebo, flunitrazepam 1 mg and triazolam 0.25 mg have been shown to impair stimulus encoding and memory-scanning/serial comparison stages of information processing both 1 h and 10 h following treatment, while the same drugs have little effect on response-selection organisation. No impairment at any of the stages was found following lormetazepam 1 mg.

## References

Atkinson RC, Shiffrin RM (1971) The control of short-term memory. Scientific American 224:82–90

Bixler EO, Scharf MB, Kales A (1972) Drugs and Sleep: effects of drugs on sleep stages, mood and performance and effectiveness of drugs in inducing and maintaining sleep. N.A.T.O. Symposium: Aviemore mimeograph

Bixler EO, Scharf MB, Soldatos CR, Mitsky DJ, Kales A (1979) Effects of hypnotic drugs on memory. Life Sci 25:1379–1388

Clarke PRF, Eccersley PS, Frisby JP, Thornton JA (1970) The amnesic effect of diazepam (Valium). Br J Anaesth 42:690–697

Dundee JW, George DA (1976) The amnesic action of diazepam, flunitrazepam and lorazepam in man. Acta Anaesthesis Belg 27:3–11

Haffner JFW, Mørland J, Setekleiv J, Strømsaether CE, Danielsen A, Frivif PT, Dybing F (1973) Mental and psychomotor effects of diazepam and alcohol. Acta Pharmacol Toxicol 32:161

Heisterkamp DV, Cohen PJ (1975) The effect of intravenous premedication with lorazepam (Ativan), pentobarbitone or diazepam on recall. Br J Anaesth 47:79–81

Hindmarch I (1976) A sub-chronic study of the subjective quality of sleep and psychological measures of performance on the morning following nighttime medication with temazepam. Arzneim Forsch/Drug Res 26:2113–2116

Klatzky RL (1980) Human Memory. Freeman, San Francisco

Liljequist R, Mattila MJ (1979) Acute effects of temazepam and nitrazepam on psychomotor skills and memory. Acta Pharmacol Toxicol (Kbh) 44:364–369

McKay AC, Dundee JW (1980) Effect of oral benzodiazepines on memory. Br J Anaesth 52:1247–1257

Mørland J, Setekleiv J, Haffner JFW, Strømsaether CE, Danielsen A, Wethe GH (1974) Combined effects of diazepam and ethanol on mental and psychomotor functions. Acta Pharmacol Toxicol 34:5

Roth T, Piccione P, Salis P, Kramer M, Kaffeman M (1979) Effects of temazepam, flurazepam and quinalbarbitone on sleep: Psychomotor and cognitive function. Br J Clin Pharmacol 8:47–54

Rundell OH, Williams HL, Lester BK (1977) Comparative effects of alcohol, secobarbital, methaqualone and meprobamate on information processing and memory. In: Gross MM (ed) Alcohol intoxication and withdrawal III a: Biological aspects of ethanol. Plenum, New York, pp 617–628

Rundell OH, Williams HL, Lester BK (1978) Secobarbital and information processing. Percept Mot Skills 46:1255–1264

Seppälä T, Dreyfus JF, Saario I, Nuotto E (1982) Zoplicone and flunitrazepam in healthy subjects: Hypnotic activity, residual effects on performance and combined effects with alcohol. Drugs Exp Clin Res 8(1):35–47

Siegfried K, Koeppen D, Taeuber K, Badian M, Malerczyzyk V, Sittig W (1981) A double-blind comparison of the acute effects of clobazam and lorazepam on memory and psychomotor functions. In: Hindmarch I, Stonier PD (eds) Clobazam. Royal Society Medicine, London

Sperling G (1960) The information available in brief visual presentations. Psychol Monogr 74(11):1– 29

Sternberg S (1969) Memory scanning: Mental processes revealed by reaction time experiments. Am Sci 57:421–457

Subhan Z (1981) A dose-range comparison of clobazam and diazepam: II. Effects on memory. In: Hindmarch I, Stonier PD (eds) Clobazam. Royal Society Medicine, London

Subhan Z (1982) The effects of benzodiazepines on short-term memory capacity. In: Benzodiazepines, sleep and daytime performance. Medicine Publishing Foundation, Oxford

Williams HL, Rundell OH, Landgrave TS (1981) Dose effects of secobarbital in a Sternberg Memory Scanning Task. Psychopharmacology (Berlin) 72:161–165

# Simulated Car Driving as a Useful Technique for the Determination of Residual Effects and Alcohol Interaction After Short- and Long-Acting Benzodiazepines

H. P. Willumeit[1], H. Ott[2] and W. Neubert[1]

**Contents**



**Abstract**

*Subjects and methods:* 54 healthy volunteers took part in 3 placebo controlled double-blind trials designed partly as crossover, partly as parallel group studies. The long-acting (elimination half-life > 24 h) test drugs diazepam (DIA 5; 10 mg) and flurazepam (FLU 30 mg) were compared to the short-acting drugs (elimination half-life < 12 h) lormetazepam (LOR 1.5; 2 mg) and mepindolol sulfate (MEP 10 mg; betablocker) following acute or subchronic application. Alcohol (ALC; 0.4–0.8 per mill blood ALC concentration) was used as a compound interfering with the test drugs. Measurements with the driving simulator TS2 were taken at different times between 1 h and 15 h p.a.

*Results:* Subchronic use of FLU causes significant impairment of driving performance the next morning in contrast to LOR which even increases the driving ability. The ALC potentiating effect of LOR is larger than that of DIA after acute intake. MEP acts like placebo but reduces blood pressure and heart rate. Interaction of LOR and ALC in the evening does not result in a prolonged hangover effect which could disturb driving performance the next morning.

*Discussion:* Short-acting benzodiazepines without active metabolites have a profound advantage over those with long-acting accumulating characteristics in respect to matutinal car driving ability, if those drugs are used as nighttime hypnotics. These results highlight the necessity of screening hypnotic and tranquilizing drugs concerning their influence on car driving performance at different times after intake and under conditions of interactions with psychotropic drugs, especially alcohol. In view of future methodological requirements a revised model of driving simulation is presented. It is based on a coherent description of the system "driver-vehicle environment" at the level of visual conditions, vehicle behaviour and driver performance. Preliminary data are shown.

**Key Words**

Alcohol/Circulatory parameters/Control theory/Diazepam/Driving simulator/EEG/EOG/Evoked potentials/Flurazepam/Lormetazepam/Mepindolol sulfate/Oxazepam/Reaction time/Sensomotoric abilities/System "driver-vehicle-environment"/Visual analogue scales/Visual pattern processing.

---

1 Institute of Automotive Engineering, Technische Universität Berlin, D-1000 Berlin 12, FRG
2 Research Laboratories, Section Psychometrics, Schering AG, D-1000 Berlin 65, FRG

Psychopharmacology Supplementum 1
Editors: I. Hindmarch, H. Ott and T. Roth

## 1 Introduction

The driving ability of car drivers is an essential component for accident avoidance. The vehicle per se as well as the environment influence the incidence of accidents.

Driving ability means: capability of the driver to keep a technically safe vehicle on a safe road without accident and free of danger for himself and for other traffic participants. That driving ability is formed by the overall state of motivation, experience, fatigue and the actual state formed by higher cognitive functions, cue perception, response selection and sensomotor functioning.

It is important to recognize that the behaviour of the driver depends upon the overall states of the environment and vehicle as well as upon the actual states the driver has to react to in terms of specific events or vehicle responses.

Our study deals with the relationship between actual and overall states of the driver, that is, driving performance and the stressors alcohol and drugs.

The large number of traffic accidents caused by "driver failure", reflected by the statistics gathered in most countries, affords the motivation for these research activities. The official statistics of the Federal Republic of Germany addresses about 75% of accidents caused by the nebulous item "driver failure".

It can be presumed that within this poorly defined class of causes fatigue as well as undetected consumption of alcohol and/or drugs may play a more important role than statistics reveal. Investigations by the University of Hamburg (Möller and Wagner 1977) have shown that in 1960 10% of accident drivers and 1976 even 21% had taken drugs within the last 24 h before the accident occurred. These figures do not prove the influence of drugs as the cause of accident but they underline the necessity to investigate the interaction of driving ability and drugs.

## 2 Method

To investigate drug effects and to obtain relevant features of driver's performance, experiments simulating actual driving should be carried out as realistic as possible. Driving tests on roads would, of course, be the best driving simulation because those results would fit best to traffic and driving conditions; the interpretation, however, is difficult because external conditions of traffic are not controllable, for instance kind and number of external stimuli, climate etc. The few reproducible results conflict with the mentioned strategy. Also, the high expense of measurement and restricted variability of dynamic parameters are disadvantages in road tests. Sometimes, it is even impossible to test the influence of drugs on driver's behaviour because of too high an accident risk.

An alternative to these typical tasks in real traffic is given by simulator tests (Fig. 1). The advantages are low expenses of measurement, simple variability of dynamic parameters, reproducibility of experimental results, and no risk in carrying out dangerous driving tasks. The deficiency of presented information and high costs for "high fidelity" simulation must be mentioned as a disadvantage. The external validity must be proven – like in all laboratory investigations.

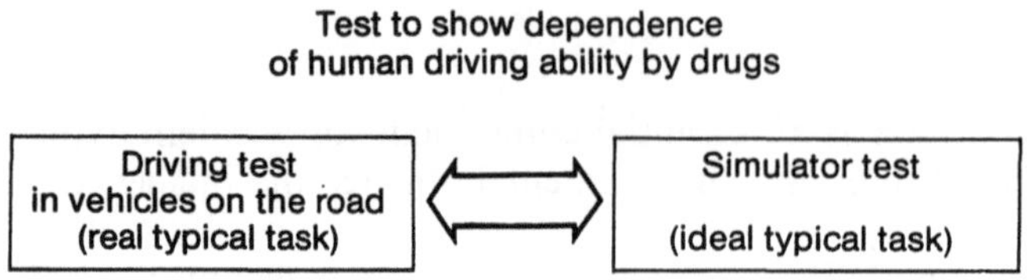


**Fig. 1.** Scheme to show dependence of human driving ability by drugs

Due to the given statements the main requirements for a driving simulator with respect to real driving conditions are:

- The primary task of the driver is to continuously keep the vehicle on roads with stochastic curvature.
- The secondary task of the driver is to react to rarely occurring external signals, given for instance by sudden obstacles.

These requirements for a driving simulator can be realized by a primary visual continuous control tracking task with stochastic command signals in addition to a secondary reaction task.

Our driving tracking simulator TS2 is a facility to test human sensomotor abilities, influenced by various stressors like climate, monotony, mechanical vibration, acoustics and visual stimuli as well as drugs.

Figure 2 in its upper part shows a common car on a curved road. The vehicle dynamics separate two different courses, the ideal vehicle course, given only by geometric road parameters, and the real vehicle course, influenced by road parameters as well as by the driving control activities at the steering wheel and by the dynamic behaviour of the car itself. The driver's control activities have to reflect the road condition as well as the vehicle dynamic behaviour in order to minimize the accident risk in veering off the road.

In the middle part of Fig. 2 the curvature of the vehicle course for the above driving situation is shown. The ideal curvature of the driving course during the change from a left to a right curve under ideal vehicle behaviour is shown as a dotted line and the full line marks the curvature of the vehicle course influenced by driver and vehicle for a given change in the road course. In order to avoid veering off the road and risking an accident the real curvature of the vehicle's course has to move within a certain time between the two border lines. This time space and the border lines define an admissible window for the curvature of the vehicle course. If the curvature exceeds this window the car driver risks an accident.

In the lower part of Fig. 2 the visual display of the TS2 simulator can be seen. The upper row of 37 lamps presents the command signal as the ideal curvature of the vehicle course, and the lower row of 37 lamps displays the actual curvature of the vehicle course which is almost proportional to the angle of the steering wheel but superimposed with the dynamics of the vehicle's behaviour at high speeds for lane changing manoeuvres.

In the left and right lower edges of the TS2 display, two lamps are seen which serve as visual signals for the secondary reaction task.

The subjects in front of that visual display (Fig. 3) have to react to the command signal on the upper row of lamps by moving the steering wheel. A maxi-

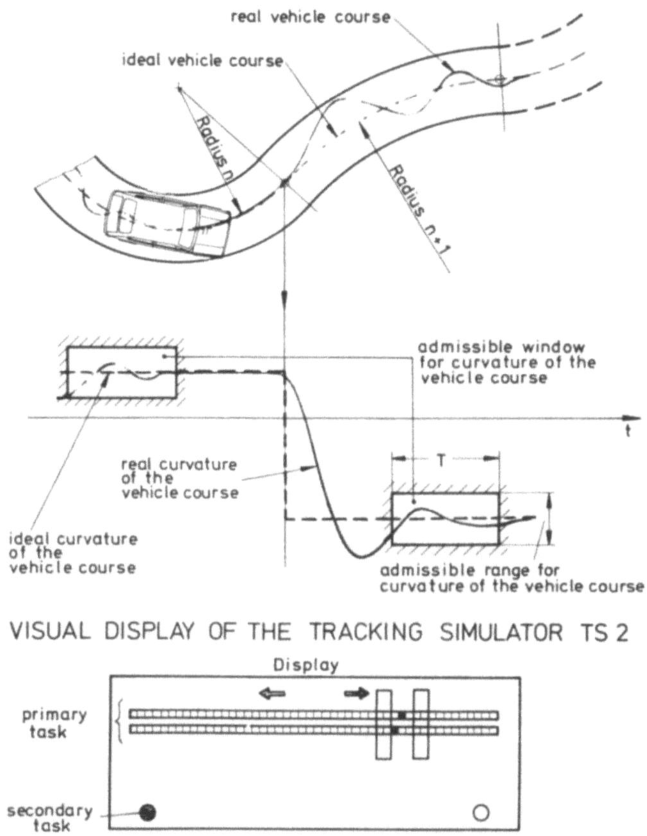


**Fig. 2.** The tracking simulator showing the ideal driving course and the visual display

mum time of 2.8 s is allowed for this task. If the subject succeeds in matching the light signals of both rows of lamps in a shorter period (admissible curvature of the vehicle course window) another task will be provided. Apart from this primary task activities the subjects have to stop the flashing of one or two extra lamps by pressing the respective pedal (left pedal if left light flashes, right pedal if right light flashes) or neither pedal if both lights flash simultaneously. That reaction time test serves as secondary task.

Figure 4 shows the typical relative decrease in the number of successfully completed primary control tasks and the typical increase of reaction times in the secondary reaction tasks for 12 subjects under the influence of 0,8 BAL (ethyl alcohol), that is the admissible limit of BAL in Germany. These results also prove the sensitivity of the simulator TS2 in respect of changes in the driver's performance and reaction time.

This simulator TS2 is a test facility which approximates actual visumotoric continuous tracking tasks and rarely occurring reaction tasks of normal car driving.

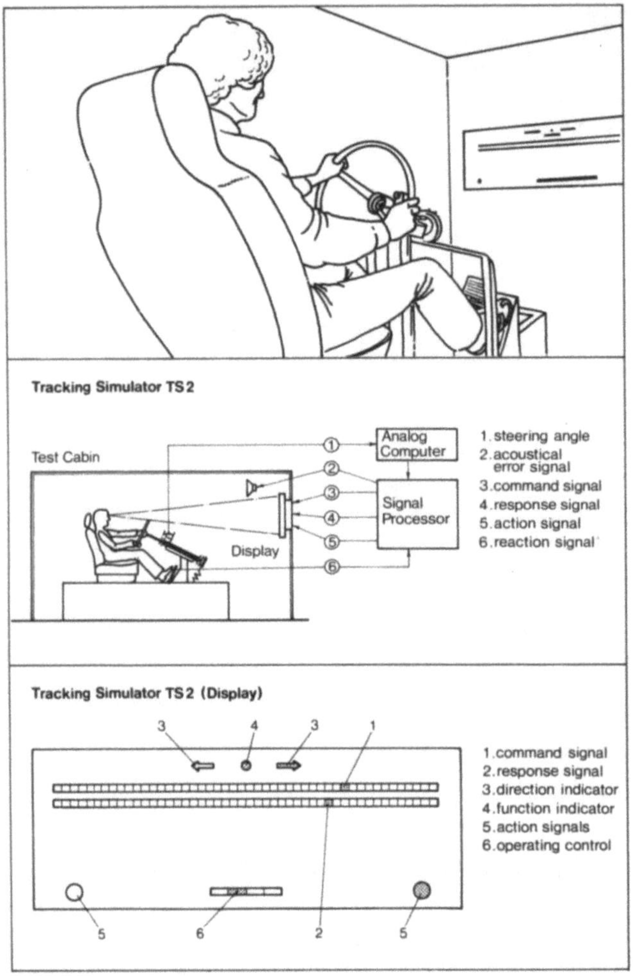


**Fig. 3.** Driving simulator TS2

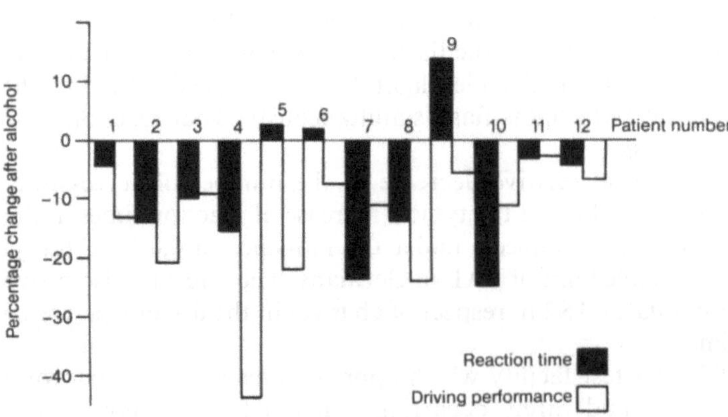


**Fig. 4.** Influence of alcohol on control tasks and reaction time for 12 subjects

## 3 Results from Different Drug Investigations

Selected from various studies results in driver's performance and reaction time are presented. The simulator tests were performed following acute or subchronic application of long-acting and short-acting drugs as well. Alcohol was used as an agent interfering with the test drugs.

In a controlled double-blind trial, designed as a crossover study, the driver's performance, reaction time and heart rate were tested following subchronic application of the short-acting drug lormetazepam (Noctamid® 2 mg, elimination half-life < 12 h), long-acting drug flurazepam (Dalmadorm® 30 mg, elimination half-life > 24 h) versus placebo. The drugs were applied to 12 healthy volunteers over a period of seven days followed by the simulator test in the morning.

The driving performance under lormetazepam (Fig. 5) shows more successfully completed tracking control tasks (2.6%) than under placebo, whereas under flurazepam the number of successfully completed control tasks is markedly reduced (− 7.26%) as compared to placebo, which implies less safe driving performance.

Obviously, the night's sleep prior to testing was positively influenced by the short-acting lormetazepam so that the driving performance was slightly superior to placebo.

The results of the driver's reaction time were slightly better under placebo (1,95%) than under lormetazepam but evidently worse (5,84%) under the long-acting flurazepam.

The heart rate was somewhat accelerated under both benzodiazepine medications.

A further controlled double-blind trial was designed as an eightfold crossover study. Lormetazepam 2 mg (Noctamid®), diazepam 10 mg (Valium®), mepindolol sulfate 10 mg (β-blocker) combined with 0,6 BAL ethyl alcohol were applied to 16 healthy subjects and tested in three courses immediately following applica-

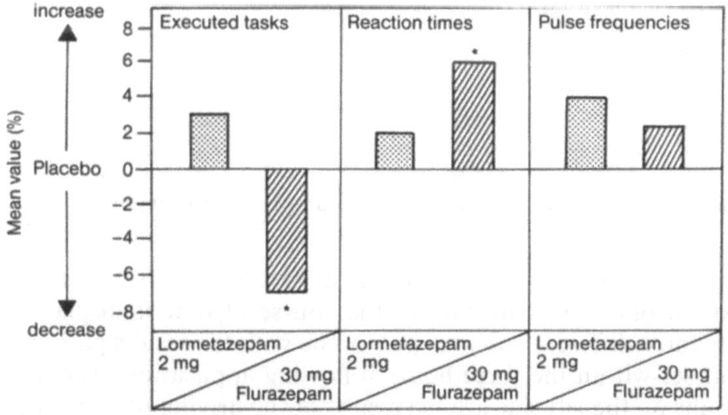


**Fig. 5.** Differences between relative changes after lormetazepam or placebo and flurazepam or placebo for 12 subjects, $*p < 0.10$

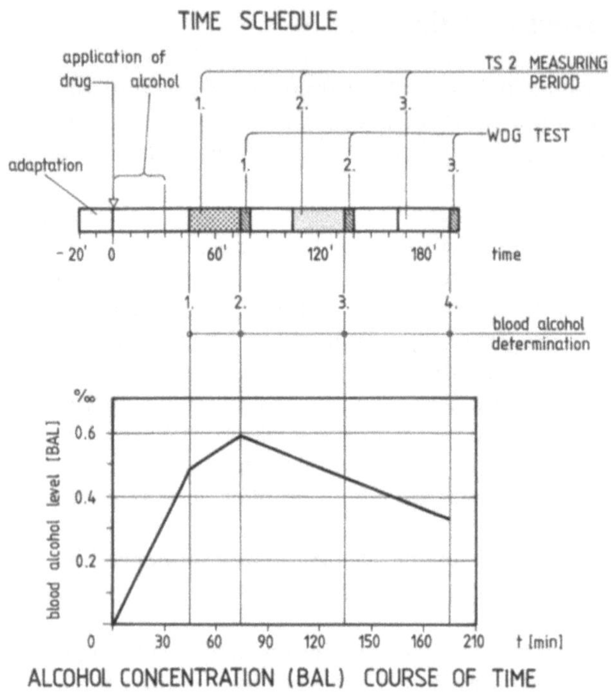


**Fig. 6.** Time schedule of tests and average BAL of subjects

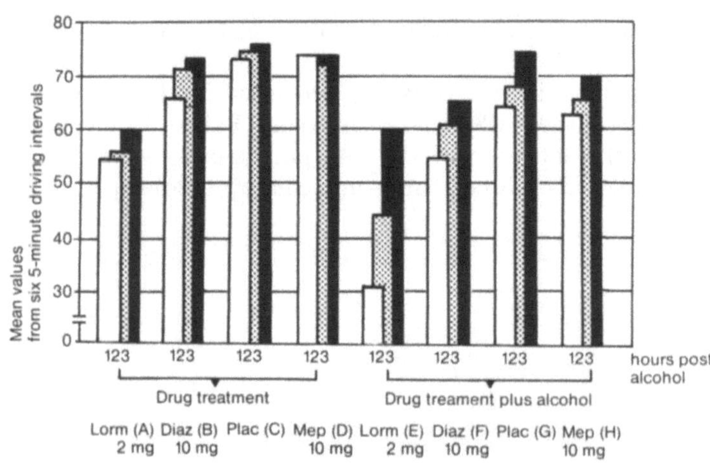


**Fig. 7.** Driving performance and number of correctly executed tasks for 16 subjects

tion. In the upper part of Fig. 6 the time schedule of measurements and in the lower part the blood alcohol concentration in the course of time is displayed.

Figure 7 presents three different columns put in line with the results gathered during the three courses within the three hours following application. The first four groups of columns on the left side are the results of the driving performance or successfully completed tracking tasks under medication without alcohol. The four groups on the right side present the results under medication plus alcohol.

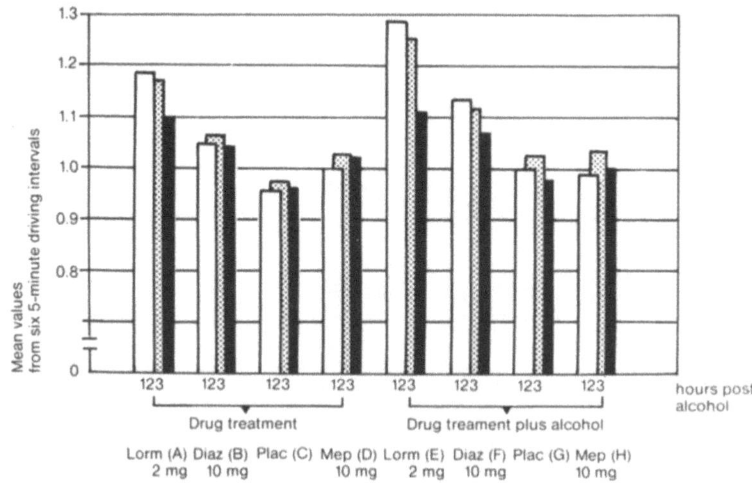


**Fig. 8.** Reaction times at driving simulator for 16 subjects

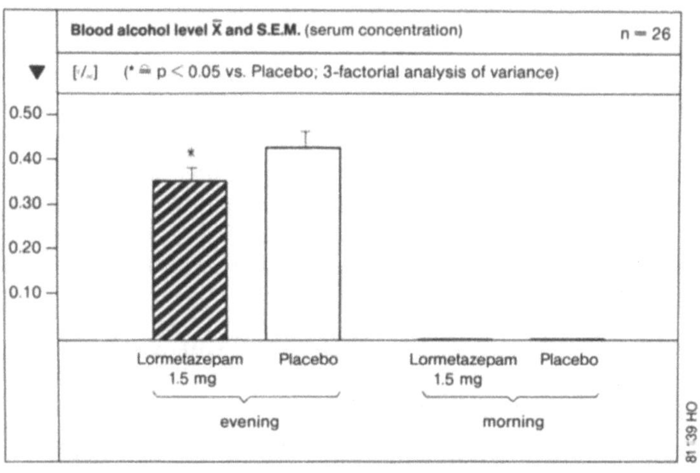


**Fig. 9.** BAL following acute intake and after 8.5 h of sleep

The effect of alcohol in combination with these medications leads to a more marked decrease in the driving performance as compared to the uncombined use of alcohol. Particularly the acute combination of alcohol and lormetazepam potentiates the effect of alcohol in reducing the driving performance but, on the other hand, leads to an evident improvement concurrently with decreasing alcohol concentrations. The combination of diazepam and alcohol reduces driving performance much more than alcohol alone.

Lormetazepam and diazepam, both with and without alcohol, have extended the reaction time as compared to placebo (Fig. 8).

A third study was conducted to test the effect on matutinal driving ability following the acute application of lormetazepam 1,5 mg as a nighttime hypnotic

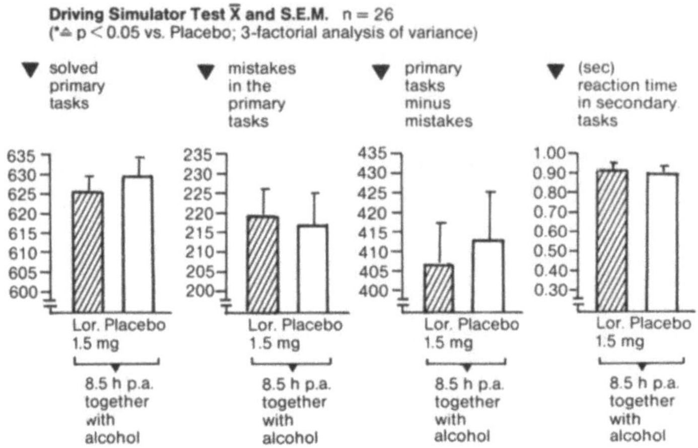


**Fig. 10.** Matutinal driving performance and reaction time after medication of 1,5 mg lormetazepam or placebo combined with alcohol in the evening

together with an alcoholic concentration of about 0,4 per mill (BAL) which mimics the probable use in actual circumstances. 26 healthy volunteers took part in a controlled double-blind trial, designed as parallel groups. The subjects took their dinner between 8.00 and 9.30 in the evening with beer or wine, followed by the application of the drug. In the evening the BAL in both groups was about 0,4 per mill and in the following morning decreased to zero as demonstrated in Fig. 9. After 8,5 h of controlled sleeping-time in the laboratory the tests were conducted.

Figure 10 shows that under these conditions no significant differences in driving performance and reaction time emerge as compared to placebo.

## 4 Discussion of the Results Based on the TS2-Simulator Tests

From the results of the studies the following conclusions may be drawn:

1) The subchronic use of flurazepam (Dalmadorm®) causes a significant impairment of driving performance in the morning whereas lormetazepam (Noctamid®) does not influence this parameter but, on the contrary, even improves the driving ability.
2) The alcohol potentiating effect of lormetazepam (Noctamid®) is higher than that of diazepam (Valium®) following acute intake.
3) Interaction of lormetazepam (Noctamid®) and alcohol in the evening does not cause prolonged hangover affecting driving performance the next morning.
4) Short-acting benzodiazepines without active metabolites have a profound advantage compared to those with protracted accumulating characteristics concerning the matutinal car driving ability when used as nighttime hypnotics.

These results highlight the necessity of screening hypnotic and tranquilizing drugs with due regard to their influence on car driving performance at different occasions, especially in combination with alcohol or other psychotrophic agents likely to cause drug interactions.

## 5 Further Methodological Developments

Whereas the driving simulator models used in the previous studies have been oriented toward the control-theory, a more recent model is geared to the principles of human visual pattern processing, since driving is primarily a complex process involving visumotor coordination.

The previously used parameters of the control-theoretical analysis were the recovery time, extent of the overshoot and complex reaction time.

The new revised model involves the analysis of eye movements in addition, whereby the subject has to cope with situations on the road viewed from a driver's perspective. At the same time the EOG (electroculogram) and two leads of the EEG ($F_4-C_z'$; $O_2-C_z''$) are recorded, allowing to take an average of the EEG segments triggered by the EOG. EEG segments are triggered by the saccadic movements following the continous changes of the visual tasks and not as a result of signal changes effected by the visual tasks themselves. This kind of EEG signals are known as lambda waves (Yagi 1979).

Pilot studies support the notion that the EEG segments, when derived in such a way, resemble the patterns of evoked potentials. In a double-blind investigation of oxazepam and placebo it was possible to isolate signal parameters which discriminated different treatments. Figure 11 presents data from an individual

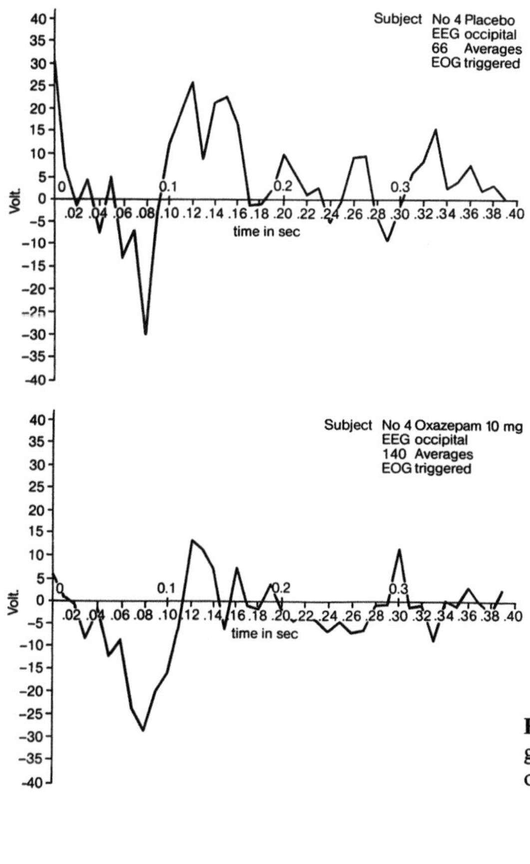


**Fig. 11.** Averaged EEG segments triggered by EOG saccadic under medication of 10 mg oxazepam or placebo

exposed to placebo and a single oral dose of 10 mg oxazepam. The upper part discloses a negative wave of approx. 80 ms and a positive wave of approx. 120 ms resulting from an average of 66 EEG segments. The lower part demonstrates the effect of oxazepam in reducing the amplitude of P120 dramatically.

It appears that the model used is adequate on the grounds that it offers a valid description of the system "driver-vehicle-environment" at the level of visual conditions, vehicle and driver behaviour. The view can be influenced by the driver's steering activities at any stage. Each parameter of the model including those of the electrophysiological variables can be reconstructed at any single stage of the trial. A more detailed description of the model is provided in a separate paper (Willumeit et al. 1983).

## References

Möller MR, Wagner HJ (1977) Über Ausmaß und Nachweis von Arzneimitteleinfluß bei Kraftfahrern. 3. Internationaler Kongreß für Verkehrsmedizin, Wien, 3.–6. 11. 1977. Institut für Rechtsmedizin der Universität des Saarlandes

Willumeit HP, Kramer U, Rohr G (1983) Closed-loop simulation of the driver-vehicle-road system. Vehicle System Dynamics 12: 141–145

Yagi A (1979) Lambda waves associated with offset of saccades: A subject with large lambda waves. Biol Psychol 8: 235–239

# Résumé

# Sleep, Benzodiazepines and Performance: Issues and Comments

I. Hindmarch[1] and H. Ott[2]

**Contents**



## 1 Introduction

In writing this overview of the verbal exchange which followed the oral presentation of the previous 16 papers we are presenting our understanding of the issues, comments, opinions, criticisms and ideas raised in debate.

An important caveat must be entered when considering the comments relating to the comparative effects of benzodiazepine hypnotics on sleep and subsequent daytime performance. The effects of benzodiazepines, or any psychoactive drug, are dependent upon the treatment regimen and dose employed, the route of administration and the sex, age and clinical characteristics of the study population. Furthermore, differences in design and statistical methodologies, assessment measures used and timing of psychometric tests must be taken account of when comparing the results of different clinical and experimental studies.

Such considerations do not preclude the validity of some of the generalizations that are made. The complexity and interactive nature of the information available on benzodiazepines, sleep and performance enforces some degree of parsimony, if a conceptualization of the whole area of debate is to be realised.

## 2 Criteria for Classifying Sleep Disorders

Approximately 20% of the general population complain of insomnia, but only 4% reach a medical setting according to prevalence studies. The absolute preva-

1 Human Psychopharmacology Research Unit, University of Leeds, GB-Leeds LS2 9JT, England
2 Research Laboratories, Section Psychometrics, Schering AG, D-1000 Berlin 65, FRG

Psychopharmacology Supplementum 1
Editors: I. Hindmarch, H. Ott and T. Roth

lence, however, is very difficult to establish. Duration is the most important aspect of insomnia. The most consistent pattern of sleep disturbance is not typically a sleep latency but a sleep fragmentation problem. Patients with transient insomnia far outnumber those with a chronic condition. The greater part of the adult population will experience transient insomnias at some time in their lives, e.g. due to travel, time zone shifts, work schedules, acute emotional disturbance.

The recuperative value of sleep has long been recognized. Differences in the metabolism of poor sleepers suggest that they have greater obstacles to recovery during sleep and may need more sleep, but get less, than other people. In experimentally induced severe acute sleep disturbances, staying awake leads to impaired physical and mental performance, coupled with a shift in the balance between synthesis and degradation of protein and reduced rates of cellular proliferative activity. The function of sleep implies an analogy to hunger and eating. The function of eating is not to relieve hunger but to provide all of those nutriments required for the sustenance of life. It may well be that the function of sleep is not to relieve sleepiness but a fulfilment of restorative demands and sleepiness is simply a signal for it.

Sleep can be measured objectively and subjectively, but important dimensions, such as the quality of sleep, have no objective determinants. All that can be ascertained are correlates of subjectively perceived sleep quality, i.e. correlations of EEG measures of total sleep time, number of awakenings etc. EEG measures of sleep onset latency, however, do not always distinguish between patients with sleep abnormalities and those without such disturbances and EEG analysis does not always discriminate between drug treatment regimens.

In individuals with "short" sleep duration there was a marked discrepancy between the number of hours they felt they had slept and the "longer" time they were objectively asleep according to EEG measures.

Some dissatisfaction with traditional scoring systems is evident, even when taking into account the attempts made to identify reasons for patients' complaints, such as micro events, e.g. number of nocturnal arousals. There is no obvious relation between traditional measures of sleep and what patients express. Likewise personality questionnaires do not adequately differentiate between "poor" and "good" sleepers.

The patient's criteria are important in clinical situations as it is the subjective complaint that leads to the prescription of hypnotics. Metabolic differences between "good" and "poor" sleepers provide evidence that the sleep of poor sleepers may indeed be less restorative. Preliminary findings indicate that hypnotics may reverse some of the detrimental metabolic concomitants of poor sleep.

Subjective criteria are a legitimate way to classify patients as "insomniacs" as they consistently complain to physicians about their sleep disturbance. When patients are evaluating their sleep, they usually refer to some aspect of the way they feel during the daytime. Sleep and nocturnal events cannot be viewed in isolation. They must always be related to daytime behaviour, as it is apparent that daytime and nighttime behaviours are complementary parts of the same circadian cycle.

One of the greatest gaps in our clinical knowledge of insomnia is what happens to a particular patient over a period of time and so it is difficult to predict for how long sleep disturbed patients should be treated, if at all. Poor sleepers might indeed be poor sleepers for the greater part of their lives and some persistent insomniacs have been known not to remit.

## 3 Withdrawal Phenomena

Withdrawal phenomena can occur on cessation of repeated dosing with benzodiazepine hypnotics. This is more associated with short, as opposed to long acting drugs. Indeed, such withdrawal phenomena rarely occur with drugs like flurazepam because of the slow elimination of active metabolites.

It is not agreed that the so-called "late night" or "early morning" insomnia is a persistent feature of withdrawal of very short acting benzodiazepines. However, objectively measured increases in early morning alertness have been found following quick acting benzodiazepine hypnotics. It cannot be determined if this "residual arousal" is the psychological sequela of a good night's sleep or directly related to the elimination of the drug from the body.

Some patients who feel "alert" in the morning following dosing with very short acting hypnotics or alcohol experience and complain of anxiety later in the day, due probably to the rapid withdrawal of the drug. In contrast benzodiazepines with long elimination half lives, i.e. in excess of 24 h, will accumulate and patients will be under the potential influence of the drug all day.

In using a hypnotic with an "intermediate" half-life, the problems of withdrawal effects are minimised. Withdrawal effects will be less severe on cessation of treatment with intermediate (8-14 h) acting drugs.

Clearly withdrawal phenomena are treatment regimen/dose related and have different frequencies of occurrence in different age groups. Recent animal and human studies with benzodiazepine antagonists support the notion that rebound effects are associated with a rapid withdrawal of the drug from the receptor sites.

## 4 Safety of the Drug

Benzodiazepines in general are well tolerated, relatively free from toxic side-effects and safe in overdose when compared to the more traditional hypnotics, e.g. barbiturates, chloral hydrate und chlormethiazole. They do, however, interact with alcohol, and other CNS depressants, which could place alcoholic patients and those receiving concurrent psychoactive medications at a greater risk of accident in car driving or social judgement situations.

There are differences between benzodiazepine hypnotics to the extent in which they influence the respiratory and cardiovascular system and to the extent in which they produce residual effects on daytime behaviour.

Serious accidents, particularly in elderly patients, have been directly attributable to the residual effects of benzodiazepine hypnotics. Grossly amnesic states, presenting as if the patients were in the early stages of senile dementia, have been reported following large doses of benzodiazepines. The amnesia resolved over a period of time on drug withdrawal, showing the direct relation between drug and amnesic potential. Lapses of memory and concentration have been reported in patient populations taking benzodiazepines. Causal as well as casual links between domestic accidents and the use of certain benzodiazepines have been established.

Patients seemingly habituate to the subjective residual effects of some hypnotics on repeated doses. Important to consider when evaluating the safety of benzodiazepine hypnotics in clinical use are the findings that objective measures of performance were impaired at times when patients perceived no ill effects. Just as sleep can only be assessed in respect of daytime behaviour, the effects of a nocturnal dose of a benzodiazepine hypnotic must be evaluated both subjectively and objectively with due regard to the residual effects it has on subsequent daytime performance.

Residual effects of benzodiazepine hypnotics are commonly measured in the early morning on risk prone activities such as car driving or on tests which are analogues of such behaviours. These measurements are meant to reflect the typical behaviours of ambulant patients who have to drive to work und use industrial machinery. However, not much attention has been paid to the residual effects on "safety test analogues" during the afternoon and evening following nocturnal medication. More research needs to be conducted on the relationship between circadian variables and the residual effects of hypnotics especially with a view to investigating the reports of "rebound anxiety" during the afternoon following the nocturnal use of some benzodiazepines.

The amnesic properties of benzodiazepines as a group are well known to anaesthetists but recent findings suggest that many benzodiazepines used as hypnotics also impair memory. The impairment is anterograde but can persist during the day following nocturnal use. Amnesia is not a simple function of the sedation produced by benzodiazepines, as short term memory deficits can be found when there is no measurable sedation.

Differences in experimental results using different memory assessment techniques can probably be explained by the relative emphasis placed on speed and/or accuracy of the subjects' response. Computer assisted information processing assessments which measure memory encoding, storage and retrieval mechanisms have distinct advantages in discriminating between benzodiazepines when compared to more traditional methods, e.g. digit span. The amnesic action of benzodiazepines has been demonstrated in numerous studies using a wide range of experimental techniques and could be explained, theoretically, by state dependent learning.

It is unlikely that residual amnesia found following the nocturnal application of some drugs is a function of sleep onset latency per se as this was not changed in some instances when amnesic effects were observed. This is not to say that sleep variables do not have some impact on the extent and nature of the amnesia produced by benzodiazepines but it is evidently secondary to a direct drug action.

Of concern in the clinical treatment of insomnia, particularly in elderly patients and others with reduced cognitive capacity, is the impairment of short term information processing which persists after the patients have wakened following the administration of a nocturnal hypnotic.

There is no evidence available as regards the chronic effects of repeated nocturnal doses of benzodiazepine hypnotics on the integrity of "long term" memory and cognitive systems, although sub-chronic studies have failed to show any habituation to amnesic properties of certain benzodiazepines.

There is no concordance between clinicians, psychologists and pharmacologists as to the theoretical definitions of, and the empirical distinctions between "recent", "short" and "long" term memory. However, it is agreed that individuals need an intact short term memory, as part of their information processing system to successfully respond to the continuous cognitive demands of everyday living.

Clinicians are increasingly recognising that their patients' complaints of "poor memory" are associated with certain drug treatment regimens. Laboratory based controlled studies have also shown that potent amnesic effects are directly and exclusively related to the psychopharmacological actions of some benzodiazepines.

## 5 Pharmacokinetics

The elimination half-life of a drug per se does not provide an adequate pharmacokinetic basis for characterising the substance. Absorption, redistribution, route of administration and galenic formulation variables are all equally important in determining the effectiveness and tolerability of the drug.

With some substances there is little agreement between different laboratories as to the range of their elimination half-lives and values of other pharmacokinetic variables. This is partly due to the different pharmacological techniques and drug treatment regimens employed by individual research groups but is more likely to be a reflection of the degree of complexity of the benzodiazepine receptors and of the inter- and intra-subject variability in the rate of their CNS adaptation.

Patients who have loaded their stomach with food and drink will delay gastric emptying and the rate of drug absorption will be significantly reduced, although the completeness of absorption will not be changed. Intravenous administration of the drug will avoid problems associated with gastro-intestinal absorption in the presence of food, but i.v. preparations are not convenient for the majority of insomniacs. Presentations of a benzodiazepine hypnotic as a suppository or in a sublingual formulation can overcome the problems of delayed absorption caused by late night eating. Benzodiazepines given in a sublingual formulation are at least as clinically effective as when given orally. Sublingual formulations are also useful in geriatric patients when difficulties in swallowing tablets are experienced.

The pharmacokinetics of benzodiazepines in clinical use are changed by both inter- und intra-patient variables. Age, sex, physical disease (especially of the kidneys and liver), concomitant medication with psychotropics, and/or alcohol and/or drugs which affect gastric absorption and eating habits and alter the rate of drug metabolism and excretion, make it difficult to identify with any degree of certainty the specific pharmacokinetic basis for observed clinical events.

The circadian rhythms of wakefulness and sleep are associated with physiological changes that modify the rate of metabolism of psychotropic drugs. This implies that benzodiazepine hypnotics will have a different pharmacokinetic profile when taken at night as compared to that usually determined from daytime experimentation. The development of radioimmunoassay techniques has promoted the understanding of the relative role played by parent compounds and their metabolites in determining the pharmacokinetic and pharmacodynamic characteristics of benzodiazepines.

## 6 Pharmacodynamics

Drugs with long elimination half-lives have a tendency to produce sedative "hangovers" the day following treatment, especially after repeated doses. However, this is not meant to imply that the shortest elimination half-life is necessarily the best criterion for examining hypnotic efficacy and tolerability. Indeed the presence, or absence, of residual amnesic effects, an important clinical aspect in the treatment of elderly insomniacs, is not related to the elimination half-life of hypnotics. In this respect drugs with "very short" and others with "very long" half-lives may, in fact, be equipotent in producing detrimental amnesic effects during the day following treatment.

Discrimination between benzodiazepine hypnotics must be made with respect to their relative durations of action which might be defined by their residual effects, such as sedation, impairment of memory, or anxiety. The pharmacodynamic action of a benzodiazepine hypnotic on a patient's cognitive behavioural, affectual and memory systems ought to be the criterion for discriminating between the various compounds, as measures of basic pharmacokinetic dimensions do not single out clinically important differences between the substances.

In order to establish the pharmacodynamic profile of a particular drug it is necessary to measure objectively the duration of action of that substance on clinically relevant variables, e.g. residual sedation, anxiogenic rebound and amnesic effects. Individual benzodiazepines have a distinct und unique profile of duration of action over different measures. Long elimination half-life drugs can be found without residual effects on memory, but equally, short elimination half-life drugs may be found to produce long lasting impairment of memory and vice versa. It is clear that such complex pharmacodynamic profiles of action are not explainable by simple pharmacokinetic variables.

## 7 Criteria for Drug Efficiency

In clinical practice the efficiency and tolerability of benzodiazepine hypnotics are determined by evaluating a patient's subjective response. On the other hand, in the sleep research laboratory, hypnotic efficiency is judged by objective EEG measures. Hypnotics are prescribed for the symptomatic relief of disturbed sleep and not as a treatment of insomnia. If patients report subjective relief following the administration of a hypnotic, that drug could be said to be effective. There are, however, many deviations from this rule as, for example, some patients report placebo to be efficacious, even though their sleep EEG's fail to show an improvement.

The function of sleep in man is not yet clear and, therefore, it is difficult to determine by which EEG measures the potency of a hypnotic is to be assessed. However, the hypnotic potential of a drug can be demonstrated using a convergent approach whereby a general improvement of subjective, correlated with improvements in objective measures should be regarded as evidence of hypnotic efficiency. Efficient hypnotics are often defined as drugs that induce and prolong sleep. There is, however, great variability in the duration of sleep in patient populations. Future hypnotics might not increase sleep duration or even the speed of sleep onset, but in some way improve the "intensity" and "restorative" quality of sleep.

Hypnotics should be well tolerated and free from sequelae which pose risks to the physical and mental well-being of the patient. A hypnotic which improves sleep without producing any untoward disturbances of behaviour the next day and is free from toxic effects, could be said to have a positive "risk/benefit ratio" and be suitable for general clinical use. An important aspect of the risk/benefit ratio is the objective determination of the residual effects of hypnotics on early morning performance and daytime activities. Hypnotics with residual effects are likely to be classed as less efficient than those free from such sequelae as any change in daytime behaviour will alter subsequent nocturnal sleep patterns.

## 8 Performance Tests

The variety of statistical models, experimental methodologies, psychometric techniques and different drug treatment regimens utilised by researchers account for the difficulties in comparing and correlating experimental results of discrete studies. There is still a place for the use of valid and reliable psychomotor tests, providing they have been shown to be sensitive to the effects of benzodiazepines in evaluating the residual action of hypnotics on performance.

Computer assisted and "on-the-road tests" of car driving have provided objective evidence of the differences between benzodiazepine hypnotics in their effects on the habitual aspect of early morning performance. The Multiple Sleep Latency Test (MSLT) has been proven to be a sensitive and reliable way of assessing the sedative action of psychotropic agents, and MSLT measures have been shown to correlate with previous night sleep variables. An increasing sophistication in the use of the pharmaco-EEG, evoked potentials and physiological techniques has enabled more precise information to be reported regarding the CNS action of benzodiazepines in both normal and patient populations.

As many benzodiazepines have an established clinical action as amnesic agents, all putative hypnotics should be screened for their residual effects on information processing and short term memory functions. Future psychometric assessments of sleep and the residual effects of benzodiazepines should always attempt to link nocturnal and daytime behaviours as complementary aspects of the same cyclic phenomenon.

Common methodologies and research designs would greatly facilitate international research efforts and contribute to the establishment of a corpus of agreed information on the relative effectiveness and risk/benefit ratios of the available benzodiazepine hypnotics.

## 9 The Ideal Hypnotic

There may not, in general, be an ideal hypnotic. The individual demands of a particular patient might be well suited by a drug which is not tolerated by another. The change in symptomatology during the course and duration of an episode of sleep disturbance may necessitate a change in medication. A chronic insomniac might have different criteria for defining an ideal hypnotic when compared to those made by a transiently sleep disturbed patient. The elderly are different from the young on important pharmacokinetic and pharmacodynamic dimensions, suggesting different treatment schedules to be employed in old and young insomniacs. An effective hypnotic will be ideal for particular patient groups, and greater specificity of prescribing regimens for different clearly defined age/treatment groups need to be made.

## 10 Anxiety/Alertness

Anxiety has a direct effect on sleep and can be one of the symptoms associated with sleep disturbance. The administration of a sedative benzodiazepine during the day for its anxiolytic effects could well augment the sleep disturbance and post daytime problems for patients via impairment of psychomotor skills.

As performance potential and anxiety levels are related, it is theoretically possible for benzodiazepine hypnotics with residual effects on anxiety to either improve or impair an individual's performance. However, it must be remembered that sedation is an intrinsic property of the 1,4-benzodiazepine molecule, and residual *sedative* sequelae involve a greater risk for daytime safety and subsequent nocturnal behaviour than the small changes in daytime anxiety/performance levels produced by some drugs.

## 11 Adaptation and Habituation

There is evidence that patients adapt to the daytime sleepiness and sedation produced by some hypnotics following repeated nocturnal dosing over prolonged periods of time, but the effects of these drugs on sleep do not show signs of habituation. There are two components to adaptation, an anxiolytic and a hypnotic one, which could be reflections of the profile of benzodiazepine action. It is important to remember that adaptation may occur at all levels from the receptor site in the CNS to the behaviour of patients taking the drugs. Behavioural as well as psychophysiological and pharmacological habituation must be considered in explaining adaptation to the effects of benzodiazepine hypnotics.

There is a known proportional relationship between the concentration of a benzodiazepine hypnotic in the blood and that at the receptor site. As a consequence, the time course of action of drugs and their metabolites at the receptor can be ascertained and predictions made about pharmacodynamic CNS changes from a consideration of blood concentrations.

Based on the evidence available, it is presumed that the more the receptor adapts to the presence of a drug, the greater will be the consequences of the drug's removal. Repeated doses of a drug produce greater quantitative changes in the sensitivity of CNS receptors than acute doses, but there is no proof of accumulation either of active substance or of metabolites to explain these changes in sensitivity. Receptor kinetics are complex – a decrease in receptor sensitivity, i.e. "down-regulation" with repeated dosage has been suggested to explain habituation phenomena. Animal studies, on the one hand, failed to demonstrate any change in receptor sensitivity following repeated drug administration. On the other hand, objective measures of daytime sedation on patients having received chronic doses of benzodiazepines for two years showed no signs of sleepiness whereas acute doses of the same benzodiazepines were found to be particularly potent in producing daytime tiredness and sedation. Such evidence suggests that there is, at least, a habituation to some of the residual effects of benzodiazepine hypnotics.

# Author Index

Page numbers in *italics* refer to the References

# Subject Index

FSC
www.fsc.org
MIX
Papier aus verantwortungsvollen Quellen
Paper from responsible sources
FSC® C105338

If you have any concerns about our products, you can contact us on
**ProductSafety@springernature.com**

In case Publisher is established outside the EU, the EU authorized representative is:
**Springer Nature Customer Service Center GmbH**
**Europaplatz 3, 69115 Heidelberg, Germany**

Printed by Libri Plureos GmbH
in Hamburg, Germany